RT82 £33.92

(QV 448)

D0726181

The Advanced Practice Registered Nurse as a Prescriber

Marie Annette Brown
PhD, ARNP, FNP-BC, FAAN
Professor
University of Washington
Seattle, WA
Primary Care Nurse Practitioner
Women's Health Care Clinic
University of Washington Medical Center
Seattle, WA

Louise Kaplan
PhD, ARNP, FNP-BC, FAANP
Director of Nursing
St. Martin's University
Lacey, WA

WILEY-BLACKWELL

A John Wiley & Sons, Inc., Publication

This edition first published 2012 © 2012 by John Wiley & Sons, Ltd.

Wiley-Blackwell is an imprint of John Wiley & Sons, formed by the merger of Wiley's global Scientific, Technical and Medical business with Blackwell Publishing.

Registered office: John Wiley & Sons Ltd, The Atrium, Southern Gate, Chichester, West Sussex, PO19 8SQ, UK

Editorial offices: 2121 State Avenue, Ames, Iowa 50014-8300, USA
The Atrium, Southern Gate, Chichester, West Sussex, PO19 8SQ, UK
9600 Garsington Road, Oxford, OX4 2DQ, UK

For details of our global editorial offices, for customer services and for information about how to apply for permission to reuse the copyright material in this book please see our website at www.wiley.com/wiley-blackwell.

Library of Congress Cataloging-in-Publication Data

Brown, Marie Annette.
  The advanced practice registered nurse as a prescriber /
Marie Annette Brown, Louise Kaplan.
    p. ; cm.
  Includes bibliographical references and index.
  ISBN-13: 978-0-8138-0524-5 (pbk. : alk. paper)
  ISBN-10: 0-8138-0524-4 (pbk. : alk. paper)
  I. Kaplan, Louise. II. Title.
  [DNLM: 1. Advanced Practice Nursing. 2. Drug Prescriptions–nursing.
  3. Pharmaceutical Preparations–administration & dosage. WY 128]
      LC classification not assigned
          615.1'4–dc23
            2011031409

A catalogue record for this book is available from the British Library.

Wiley also publishes its books in a variety of electronic formats. Some content that appears in print may not be available in electronic books.

Set in 9/11 pt Palatino by Toppan Best-set Premedia Limited

Printed and bound in Malaysia by Vivar Printing Sdn Bhd

Disclaimer

To my husband, Eric Leberg, whose deeply loving support has inspired and sustained me. To my patients, students, and colleagues who have fueled my enthusiasm for a lifelong dedication to the advanced practice nursing role. And to my father, Moss Brown, who led me to the understanding that education is transformative.

Marie Annette Brown

To my sons, Kai and Lee, for their understanding of the time I spent working on this project and advocating for advanced practice registered nurses. And to all the advanced practice registered nurses who have worked tirelessly to further autonomous practice nationwide.

Louise Kaplan

Contents

Companion website

This book is accompanied by a companion website:

www.wiley.com/go/brownandkaplan

Contents

Contributors

Editors

Marie Annette Brown, PhD, ARNP, FNP-BC, FAAN
Professor
University of Washington
Seattle, WA
Primary Care Nurse Practitioner
Women's Health Care Clinic
University of Washington Medical Center
Seattle, WA

Louise Kaplan PhD, ARNP, FNP-BC, FAANP
Director of Nursing
St. Martin's University
Lacey, WA

Contributors

Carolyn Buppert, CRNP, JD
Attorney
Bethesda, MD

Nancy J. Crigger, PhD, MA, ARNP, BC
Associate Professor of Nursing
Graceland University
Independence, MO

Pamela Stitzlein Davies, MS, ARNP
Nurse Practitioner
Palliative & Supportive Care Service
Seattle Cancer Care Alliance
Seattle, WA

Elizabeth K. Kessler, MSN, APRN, FNP-C
Assistant Professor of Nursing
William Jewell College
Liberty, MO

Tracy Klein, PhD, FNP, FAANP
Advanced Practice Consultant
Oregon State Board of Nursing
Portland, OR

Elissa Ladd, PhD, RN, FNP-BC
Associate Professor
MGH Institute of Health Professions
Boston, MA

Donna Poole, MSN, ARNP, PMHNP-BC
Medical Services Manager and Psychiatric Nurse Practitioner
Kitsap Mental Health Services
Bremerton, WA

Mary Sobralske, PhD, ARNP
Certified Family Nurse Practitioner
Certified Transcultural Nurse
Transcultural Health Consultants
Spokane, WA

Preface

The purpose of this book is to provide advanced practice registered nurses (APRNs) with the information necessary to be a fully informed, rational, and ethical prescriber. The genesis of this book was our teaching, practice, and research. Throughout our professional life as nurse practitioners, we have experienced the demands and difficulties inherent in accomplishing this goal.

In 2001, Washington State APRNs obtained prescriptive authority for Scheduled II–IV drugs. Our research revealed that when this was initially optional, many APRNs did not obtain this hard-won prescriptive authority and some were reluctant to prescribe or provide these drugs. The slower-than-expected transition prompted our desire to create a more in-depth understanding of how APRNs adopt the role of a prescriber. Likewise, our colleagues, the chapter authors, were inspired to share their prescribing wisdom gleaned from experience to mentor students and colleagues. They dedicated countless days to the time-consuming and often difficult challenge of writing in addition to their ongoing professional demands.

We intend for this book to assist students who are adopting the role of APRN prescriber. We also intend to assist practicing APRNs who confront challenges as they transition to the full scope of the prescriber role. Most APRNs need to deepen their knowledge base as they fully implement new or expanded roles, particularly that of fully autonomous prescriber. Ultimately, this information will assist our colleagues across the nation as they work to advance the profession in order to serve patients. Enhancing the prescribing expertise of APRNs will enrich our professional opportunities to contribute to greater access and more patient-centered care. This expertise is also a basis on which we can create changes necessary to improve the quality of health care delivered to Americans.

In 2010, the Institute of Medicine released the report, *The Future of Nursing: Leading Change, Advancing Health*. The first key message of this report is that nurses should practice to the full extent of their education and expertise. The report recommended that legal and regulatory barriers to APRN practice be eliminated. We thank the APRNs who have worked tirelessly over the decades to do just that.

We acknowledge policymakers as well as local, state, and national nursing organizations that have been instrumental in advancing the profession of nursing. They honored the dream of advanced practice nursing pioneers who championed their creative innovation that is part of our professional heritage. We dedicate this book to the APRNs who continue the work needed to eliminate the barriers to fully autonomous prescribing for all APRNs. We will not rest until we meet that goal!

Marie Annette Brown and Louise Kaplan

The Advanced Practice Registered Nurse as a Prescriber

What Do APRN Prescribers Need to Understand?

Marie Annette Brown and Louise Kaplan

Today's health care transformations herald unprecedented opportunities for advanced practice registered nurses (APRNs) to provide and model patient-centered, evidence-based health care. As APRNs across the country secure fully autonomous practice, they must also seize the opportunity to become pacesetters for ethical and responsible prescribing. The vast majority of APRNs (nurse practitioners, nurse midwives, nurse anesthetists, and clinical nurse specialists) work with prescription medications on a daily basis. Many are unable to imagine a practice that does not, in some way, include the ability to prescribe, provide, and/or manage medications for at least some of their patients. A goal of most APRNs, however, is utilization of a wide range of healing therapies in the process of patient-centered care. This may include, but is not focused solely on medications. Health promotion and disease prevention continue to be a hallmark of APRN practice.

At the same time, as the demand for prescriptive medications increases, prescriptive authority becomes an even more vital component of APRN practice. The number of prescriptions increased 39% between 1999 and 2009 from 2.8 billion to 3.9 billion. During this same time period, the U.S. population grew only 9% (Kaiser Family Foundation, 2010). In order to meet the prescribing needs of patients, APRNs must have unencumbered and fully autonomous prescriptive authority and practice.

Practice in today's complex, fast-paced healthcare delivery system in which there is a constant barrage of information can be

The Advanced Practice Registered Nurse as a Prescriber, First Edition. Marie Annette Brown, Louise Kaplan.
© 2012 John Wiley & Sons, Ltd. Published 2012 by John Wiley & Sons, Ltd.

overwhelming. Selection and monitoring of medication appropriate for patients is only one aspect of the complex process of prescribing. This book serves as an easily accessible reference to guide practicing APRNs through these challenges and supplement pharmacotherapeutic knowledge about specific medications. APRN students can also benefit from the content of this book. Standards for APRN programs specify a pharmacotherapeutic course as well as analysis of the APRN role (National Organization of Nurse Practitioner Faculties [NONPF], 2010). Educators barely have time to teach the essential knowledge about pharmacokinetics, pharmacodynamics, and evidence-based drug treatment recommendations. There is little time available in most pharmacology courses for in-depth discussion of the APRN's role as a prescriber. The information included in this book has been compiled by experts in their areas. Each author has used her particular wisdom and creativity to synthesize and organize key ideas on a wide variety of subjects. These include:

- What it means to be a prescriber
- The many facets of the prescriber role
- The legal, regulatory, and ethical responsibilities of APRNs who prescribe medications
- Patient–APRN collaboration to reach patient-centered medication decisions
- Dealing with difficult clinical situations
- Pharmaceutical industry influences on prescriber decisions
- Cultural competencies to promote patient-centered prescribing.

THE JOURNEY OF APRN PRESCRIPTIVE AUTHORITY

For decades, APRNs have invested innumerable hours in lobbying and regulatory work to advance APRN practice. They have solidified the APRN role, strengthened the foundation for APRN education, and expanded the knowledge base for expert practice. APRNs in Idaho were the first to be authorized to prescribe medication in 1971, though it took 6 years for rules to be written and prescriptive authority to be implemented. Most APRNs have now been granted prescriptive authority in all states. APRNs have repeatedly demonstrated that they provide effective, high-quality care, including prescribing medications (Ingersoll, 2009; Newhouse et al., 2011).

Nonetheless, APRNs in nearly three-quarters of the states confront prescribing barriers on a daily basis. These barriers include requirements for supervision or collaboration, restrictions on prescribing controlled substances, and limitations on the type and quantity of medications that can be prescribed.

As a consequence of prescribing barriers, many APRNs are unable to practice to the full extent of their educational preparation, knowledge, and abilities. This negatively affects patient care and the healthcare system overall. Practice constraints handicap the APRN who is unable to fulfill roles in outpatient and inpatient settings. These restrictions continue despite an increased demand for primary, specialty and acute care providers, and the expansion of "patient-centered healthcare homes." APRNs are in more demand as work hours for medical residents have been limited and shortages of providers to work with the underserved and those living in rural areas increase. Successful implementation of healthcare reforms in the years to come requires APRNs to be full partners with other health professionals. One of the key recommendations from the Institute of Medicine's (2010) report, "The Future of Nursing: Leading Change, Advancing Health," emphasizes the need to remove barriers to allow nurses to practice to the full extent of their education and expertise.

Washington State as an exemplar

A legislature must pass a bill to enable any changes in the scope of practice for ARPNs. The law typically cannot be implemented until the Board of Nursing adopts rules that specify the intent of the law. Scope of practice changes can take months to years to finalize. The history of APRN prescribing in Washington State begins with a 1977 law that authorized advanced practice nurses to prescribe legend drugs (medications requiring a prescription). However, dispensing medications and prescribing controlled substances were prohibited. The Board of Nursing then wrote rules that authorized APRNs to prescribe Schedule V drugs in 1982 and dispensing was added in 1983. It was not until 2000, after more than a decade of lobbying, that APRNs in Washington State obtained Schedule II–IV prescriptive authority.

This long-sought authority came with a price. For the first time since APRN practice was authorized by the legislature in 1973, some type of physician involvement was mandated. APRNs who wanted II–IV prescriptive authority were required to obtain a Joint Practice Agreement (JPA) with a physician. Slowly over the next 4 years many APRNs began obtaining this type of prescriptive authority. However, until the JPA was removed, over one-third of APRNs did not obtain II–IV prescriptive authority. This contradicted the expectation of APRN leaders in the state that nearly all APRNs would want the legal ability to prescribe controlled substances even if it was only utilized occasionally. We conducted research in Washington State to understand this unexpected phenomenon (Kaplan & Brown, 2004, 2007, 2009; Kaplan, Brown, Andrilla, & Hart, 2006; Kaplan, Brown, & Donohue, 2010).

The findings of our research serve as a basis of understanding how APRNs may or may not transition to fully autonomous prescriptive authority and practice when provided the opportunity. It also offers lessons learned about the need to prepare APRNs for a major transition in scope of practice. Change may cause concern for some who have adapted to the status quo, even if prescribing barriers limited their ability to practice. Many of these findings are discussed in Chapter 3 on prescribing barriers. They will enhance your understanding about APRN prescribing practice, the consequences of limiting APRN practice, and the poorly understood experience of scope of practice change. It is not surprising, however, that APRNs respond to change with the natural ambivalence that accompanies most change processes.

OVERVIEW OF CHAPTERS

Chapter 2 guides the reader through an analysis of the role and responsibilities of the APRN as a prescriber. The ability to independently prescribe medications symbolizes the legitimacy of APRNs. The public often perceives the prescribing role as what defines an APRN. This chapter includes an overview of the development of the APRN role and prescriptive authority, the essential nature of autonomy, and the process of transition to the prescribing role. The chapter emphasizes the shift from prescribing medication based on professional preference and tradition to rational prescribing and evidence-based practice as strategies for achieving quality patient-centered care.

With all of the factors that influence the transition of the APRN to becoming a prescriber, there is an understandable degree of uncertainty and concern about prescribing. Challenges about the transition from a role that requires administration of medications and prescribed treatments as a registered nurse to manager of care and prescriber as an APRN are delineated. Change can be a professionally invigorating challenge rather than a distressing situation. It is understandable, however, that many role transitions are characterized by uncertainty along with the excitement and promise of change.

Chapter 3 highlights the multitude of challenges and opportunities that APRNs confront when prescribing medication. Laws, regulations, policies, as well as the attitudes of other health professionals often limit prescribing. These are considered external barriers to an APRN's adoption of the prescribing role. Internal barriers also can diminish an APRN's interest in fully autonomous practice and can be overlooked when analyzing barriers to APRN prescribing. Internal barriers are invisible or unacknowledged factors within the individual APRN, including personal characteristics such as conflict avoidance or the "need to be liked." Strategies to overcome internal and external prescribing barriers are offered as a way to generate enthusiasm among APRNs for facilitating change.

Chapter 4 discusses the characteristic clinical challenges inherent in prescribing controlled substances and the strategies to address them. The use of deliberate, concrete approaches to prescribing controlled substances is a key strategy to build prescribing expertise. Topics discussed range from "universal precautions" for use with the prescription of controlled substances and the assessment and management of patients with chronic noncancer pain, to clinical guidelines, consensus statements, and practice standards for the identification of a patient who is a substance abuser. The author offers online resources, examples of useful documentation, and a comprehensive reference list to further hone skill building. Accurate definitions of terms related to drug use or misuse and their application provide a rationale for creating more skillful communication with patients around complex and sensitive issues.

Chapter 5 coaches APRNs to deal with difficult and often complex clinical situations that are inherent in human relationships and professional interactions, even among experienced and dedicated APRNs. These situations often create anxiety and may even generate anger when the APRN feels ill-prepared to deal with them. The basic tenet is that these are not *problem patients* but situations for which the APRN needs more knowledge, skill, and insight from self-reflection. Examples of these situations include dealing with patients who are or appear to be seeking controlled substances, are angry, request inappropriate care such as antibiotics for a viral infection, and who violate boundaries. One goal of the discussion is to enhance understanding of why these difficult situations develop and how they can impact patient-centered care. Specific strategies to identify difficult situations, respond to them appropriately, and build competence as a supportive and courageous APRN prescriber are discussed.

Chapter 6 describes pharmaceutical marketing and its influence on APRN prescribing. There are nationwide efforts to counter drug company influence on providers and healthcare organizations that in many instances have normalized this influence. Pharmaceutical drug promotion is directed at all prescribers through activities such as drug detailing, advertising in journals, and educational offerings. The United States is the only country besides New Zealand where direct-to-consumer advertising of drugs is allowed. Consumers are targeted by advertising on the Internet, television, and in print media.

Increased APRN awareness of drug company activities may assist in understanding the direct and indirect methods used to influence providers and consumers. Continued promotional activities to APRNs and lack of regulatory constraints must be balanced with heightened level of APRN awareness, vigilance, and ethical considerations among APRNs to assure cost-effective, evidence-based prescribing.

Chapter 7 details the laws, regulations, and professional issues that affect prescribing. These include state laws, board of nursing rules, and interprofessional constraints. Fully autonomous prescribing is contrasted with examples of restricted prescribing authority. Restrictions include the requirement for physician supervision, the need to use formularies, and the lack of authority to prescribe controlled substances.

The APRN Consensus Model was developed over several years of dialogue and negotiation by representatives of education, state boards of nursing, and professional practice organizations. Discussion of the consensus model highlights the need for standardized regulation that achieves fully autonomous practice with full prescriptive authority and universal adoption of the term

APRN. This chapter can assist APRNs across the nation to visualize and positively anticipate their future practice and prescribing.

In Chapter 8 a series of case exemplars convey important legal information for APRNs. This includes prescribing authority based on state law, federal laws on prescribing controlled substances, and the standard of care for prescribing varying classes of drugs. These exemplars highlight the role of Boards of Nursing, malpractice attorneys when a lawsuit is filed, the Drug Enforcement Administration, and government auditors who monitor nursing facilities. The purpose of this chapter is to help APRNs become savvy prescribers and avoid missteps during their career.

Chapter 9 focuses on the role of cultural competence in prescribing medications. Factors such as biological variation, race, ethnicity, primary language, literacy, socioeconomics, disabilities, and religious beliefs need to be considered by the APRN. Discussion of ethnopharmacology highlights the effect of race and ethnicity on the responses to medication, drug absorption, metabolism, distribution, and excretion. Concepts about immigration, acculturation, and assimilation that influence health beliefs and behavior will enable APRNs to understand the multiple strategies necessary for prescribing in a culturally appropriate manner.

CONCLUSION

Ultimately, this book is more than a guide and reference for building and enhancing prescribing expertise. It honors the work of APRNs who use prescriptive authority to provide comprehensive quality care. The book is a tribute to the countless number of APRNs who have worked tirelessly for fully autonomous prescriptive authority. Toward that end, we hope the book is an inspiration to students. You are the next generation of APRNs on whom we depend to join in the efforts to obtain fully autonomous prescriptive authority nationwide. We look forward to the day this is achieved.

REFERENCES

Ingersoll, G. (2009). Outcomes and performance improvement: An integrative review of research on advanced practice nursing. In A. Hamric, J. Spross, & C. Hanson (Eds.), *Advanced practice nursing: An integrative approach*. St. Louis, MO: Saunders.

Institute of Medicine. (2010). *The future of nursing: Leading change, advancing health*. Washington, DC: The National Academies Press.

Kaiser Family Foundation. (2010). Prescription drug trends. Retrieved from http://www.kff.org/rxdrugs/upload/3057-08.pdf

Kaplan, L., & Brown, M. A. (2004). Prescriptive authority and barriers to NP practice. *Nurse Practitioner*, *29*(3), 28–35.

Kaplan, L., & Brown, M. A. (2007). The transition of nurse practitioners to changes in prescriptive authority. *Journal of Nursing Scholarship*, *39*(2), 184–190.

Kaplan, L., & Brown, M. A. (2009). Prescribing controlled substances: Perceptions, realities and experiences in Washington State. *American Journal for Nurse Practitioners*, *12*(3), 44–51, 53.

Kaplan, L., Brown, M. A., Andrilla, H., & Hart, L. G. (2006). Barriers to autonomous practice. *The Nurse Practitioner*, *31*(1), 57–63.

Kaplan, L., Brown, M. A. & Donohue, J. S. (2010). Prescribing controlled substances: How NPs in Washington are making a difference. *The Nurse Practitioner*, *35*(5), 47–53.

National Organization of Nurse Practitioner Faculties. (2011). Nurse practitioner core competencies. Retrieved from http://www.nonpf.org/associations/10789/files/IntegratedNPCoreCompsFINALApril2011.pdf

Newhouse, R. P., Stanik-Hutt, J., White, K. M., Johantgen, M., Bass, E., Zangaro, G., . . . Weiner, J. P. (2011). Advance practice nurse outcomes 1990–2008: A systematic review. *Nursing Economic$*, *29*(5), 1–22.

Embracing the Prescriber Role as an APRN

Louise Kaplan, Marie Annette Brown,
Nancy J. Crigger, and Elizabeth K. Kessler

This chapter emphasizes the importance of prescriptive authority as a component of advanced practice registered nurse (APRN) practice. An overview describes the development of, and transition to, the APRN role, with an emphasis on prescribing. The framework for rational prescribing rests on knowledge of the patient, knowledge about the nature of the health problem, and treatment using evidence-based guidelines, standards of care, and strategies for promoting medication use.

The ability to independently prescribe medications symbolizes the legitimacy of advanced practice registered nurses (APRNs). The public often perceives the prescribing role as what defines an APRN. Therefore, a goal of APRNs is fully autonomous practice and professional integrity to provide comprehensive patient care (Mantzoukas & Watkinson, 2007). APRNs prescribe medications to meet societal needs, the expectations of the profession, and the needs of individual patients and families. Prescribing is a component of each of the four APRN roles: certified registered nurse anesthetist (CRNA), certified nurse-midwife (CNM), clinical nurse specialist (CNS), and nurse practitioner (NP). Prescribing is within the scope of practice for NPs and CNMs in all 50 states but is more limited for CNSs and CRNAs (National Council of State Boards of Nursing, 2010). This chapter provides information for APRNs to

The Advanced Practice Registered Nurse as a Prescriber, First Edition. Marie Annette Brown, Louise Kaplan.
© 2012 John Wiley & Sons, Ltd. Published 2012 by John Wiley & Sons, Ltd.

enhance expertise and confidence for successful adoption of the fully autonomous prescriber role.

DEVELOPMENT OF THE APRN ROLE

The APRN role began with nurse anesthetists in the late 1800s, preceding anesthesiologists by several decades. Nurse midwives became established in the United States in the early 1900s, while the CNS role evolved in the 1940s (Dunphy, Smith, & Youngkin, 2009). The NP role, developed in 1965, has grown the most rapidly, with NPs becoming the largest group of APRNs. Nationally, NP educational programs more than doubled between 1992 and 1997 (Druss, Marcus, Olfson, Tanielian, & Pincus, 2003).

During the 1980s and 1990s, many legislatures enacted laws that provided a scope of practice for APRNs consistent with their educational preparation (Hamric, Spross, & Hanson, 2009). Over time, APRNs have established themselves as members of the healthcare workforce with a distinct role, a unique education, and essential knowledge and skills to provide care.

APRN scope of practice varies across the United States according to state laws that are the basis of regulation (Pearson, 2011). Advanced practice nursing is controlled by licensure, accreditation, credentialing, and educational preparation, and practice opportunities at higher levels of expertise (Brown-Benedict, 2008; Ford, 2008; Klein, 2008). Variation in APRN roles also result from organizational policies that may support or constrain practice. APRNs are responsible for maintaining a high ethical standard in practice, generating knowledge, and appraising and translating evidence to provide quality, comprehensive, patient-centered care.

Although there has been significant progress in the utilization of APRNs, constraints on consumers' access to APRNs, legal limitations, and absence of a consistent, fully autonomous scope of practice across states continue to be problematic (Lugo, O'Grady, Hodnicki, & Hanson, 2007). Constraints on APRNs that limit their practice are not supported by data about the quality of care they provide (Fairman, Rowe, Hassmiller, & Shalala, 2011). Over the last several decades, studies have demonstrated that APRN care is as or is more effective than care given by physicians (Brown & Grimes, 1995; Congressional Budget Office, 1979; Dulisse & Cromwell, 2010; Horrocks, Anderson, & Salisbury, 2002; Laurant et al., 2006; Lenz,

Mundinger, Kane, Hopkins, & Lin, 2004; Newhouse et al., 2011; Ohman-Strickland et al., 2008; Prescott & Driscoll, 1980; Safriet, 1992; Simonson, Ahern, & Hendryx, 2007; Spitzer et al., 1974; Wright, Romboli, DiTulio, Wogen, & Belletti, 2011). Many of these studies also validated more widespread acceptance of the APRN role and high satisfaction with APRN care. Increasing demands for APRNs (Fairman et al., 2011) and assessment of their cost-effectiveness (Bauer, 2010) are expected to influence removal of legal barriers remaining in many states. Concurrently, an improved regulatory environment, especially in relationship to prescriptive authority, has helped legitimize and distinguish the APRN role. In states where NPs have fully autonomous practice, prescribing autonomously is a major difference between NPs and physician assistants (PAs) whose practice is always supervised by and is legally linked with a physician. Furthermore, implementation of the *Consensus Model for APRN Licensure, Accreditation, Certification and Education* (see Chapter 7) can assist APRNs to attain fully autonomous practice, including complete prescriptive authority.

Autonomy is an important professional concept for APRNs; the nursing literature on advanced practice confirms it has been difficult to achieve (Ulrich & Soeken, 2005; Weiland, 2008). The conceptualization of autonomy by Weiland (2008) uses both a legal definition and "…the practical ability to provide primary health care and exercise independent judgment and self-governance within the NP scope of practice" (p. 345). Autonomy is also a professional and personal sense of the ability to make decisions in practice independently when legally granted to a professional through the endorsement of society. Autonomy extends beyond the legal authorization to prescribe. "It is not just in action but in thought that we create our autonomy" (Kaplan & Brown, 2006, p. 37).

DEVELOPMENT OF THE APRN ROLE AND PRESCRIPTIVE AUTHORITY

Obtaining prescriptive authority for APRNs has presented significant challenges nationwide. Even when prescriptive authority is supported in new legislation, significant roadblocks with implementation often occur, particularly those placed by physicians. In 1971, for example, Idaho became the first state to pass legislation that recognized the NP role and granted prescriptive authority. Although the first Idaho NP entered practice in 1972, opposition from the Board of Medicine resulted in more than one dozen drafts of the prescriptive authority rules. It was not until 1977 that the rules were adopted, and Idaho became the first state to implement prescriptive authority for NPs (personal communication, S. Evans, December 28, 2009). Nearly 30 years later, in 2006, Georgia became the last state to pass a law granting APRNs authority to "order" medications, a variant of prescribing (Phillips, 2007).

As discussed in Chapter 1 and in Chapter 7, the prescribing role remains tightly controlled in many states. In only 15 states and in the District of Columbia (depending on the definition used) is there prescriptive authority for NPs without physician involvement. In the remaining states, NPs have various requirements for physician involvement when prescribing. Prescribing is within the scope of practice for CNMs in all 50 states with varying degrees of physician involvement but is more limited for CNSs and CRNAs. Nurse anesthetists can prescribe in 29 states (Kaplan, Brown, & Simonson, 2011) and CNSs in 34 states (National Council of State Boards of Nursing, 2010).

ADAPTING TO THE APRN'S ROLE AS PRESCRIBER
Prescriptive authority
Prescriptive authority is the legal ability to prescribe drugs and devices, a practice regulated by the states. One aspect of prescriptive authority, controlled substances (CSs), is specifically regulated by the federal government through the Drug Enforcement Administration (DEA) (Arcangelo & Peterson, 2006). States may also have additional regulations related to prescribing CSs.

Transition to the prescribing role
One of the greatest responsibilities for an APRN is that of prescription medication management. Prescribing is not a part of the registered nurse (RN) role, and often requires a major paradigm shift to transition from administering drugs to selecting and prescribing medications. Consequently, the individual APRN's transition to the prescriber role involves a union between knowledge of and socialization to the role. APRNs begin gaining knowledge and competencies throughout their graduate education and continue

this process through practice. Role socialization is also initiated during APRN education and will likewise be part of continuing professional development.

Transition to the prescriber role is part of the larger role transition that the APRN experiences first as a student, as a novice practitioner, and when scope of practice changes. Schumacher and Meleis (1994) identified five factors that influence role transition. These are:

1. Personal meaning of the transition
2. Degree of planning for the transition
3. Environmental barriers and supports
4. Level of knowledge and skill
5. Expectations.

Identification of these factors may allow the APRN to prepare ways for a smooth transition although there are other dimensions of transition that also need to be considered.

Students in APRN programs typically experience a role transition process that involves role confusion and role strain including tension, frustration, and anxiety. Role acquisition as a student may involve four stages of development (Brykcznski, 2009):

1. Complete dependence with a loss of confidence and feelings of incompetence
2. Developing competence, a personal practice philosophy and standards of practice, and increased confidence in the ability to succeed
3. Independence in making practice decisions with the possibility of disagreement in approaches between student and preceptor or faculty
4. Interdependence with the development of a personal vision of the APRN role and relationships with other health professionals.

Role acquisition extends to the practicing APRN. The first year of practice is an especially challenging one. A study by Brown and Olshansky (1998) identified four stages in the transition to primary care NP role. These are laying the foundation, launching, meeting the challenge, and broadening the perspective. Table 2.1 describes these stages. The study findings revealed the importance of skillful mentors who serve as a compass to guide the NP and serve as a

Table 2.1 Nurse practitioners' experience during the first year of primary care practice

Stage 1: Laying the Foundation
   Recuperating from school
   Negotiating the bureaucracy
   Looking for a job
   Worrying

Stage 2: Launching
   Feeling real
   Getting through the day
   Battling time
   Confronting anxiety

Stage 3: Meeting the challenge
   Increasing competence
   Gaining confidence
   Acknowledging system problems

Stage 4: Broadening the perspective
   Developing system savvy
   Affirming oneself
   Upping the ante

Source: Reprinted from Brown and Olshansky (1998), with permission from Wolters Kluwer Health.

source of information and support. Access to a mentor can be especially important in respect to adoption of the role of a prescriber, which brings a special set of challenges.

Grappling with questions about prescribing contribute to professional development and strengthen prescribing expertise during an APRN's career.

- What is the APRN's role in a particular healthcare setting?
- What is the APRN's relationship to a collaborating physician when this relationship is required by state law?
- How does one adapt practice when relocating to a state with a different level of restriction that provides either more or less autonomy?

General questions are often followed by more specific patient-centered questions.

- Am I making the right medication choice?
- What type of antibiotic should be prescribed to treat a methicillin-resistant *Staphylococcus aureus* infection?
- How long should I manage a patient with uncontrolled diabetes before initiating insulin therapy?

When faced with the reality of determining specific practice decisions, particularly those about prescribing, the novice APRN may experience a sense of uncertainty. Novice APRNs are also brave when they assume the APRN role. They enter into advanced practice step-by-step, decision-by-decision. Experience is a remarkable teacher, and gradually, APRNs integrate their professional practice and develop a comfort with prescribing. APRNs need time to transition into their new role. The "one-size fits-all" expectation does not apply to the APRN role which is highly variable from state to state and within individual workplace settings (Deshefy-Longhi, Swartz, & Grey, 2008).

Another aspect of adopting the APRN role is to grapple with constantly changing constraints imposed on all prescribers by health plans and healthcare delivery systems. For example, insurers promote the use of generic medications by requiring higher co-payments or refusing to pay for some brand name drugs. Healthcare systems such as the Veterans Administration (VA) or health maintenance organizations such as Kaiser Permanente increasingly use formularies. These limit the medications that are available for patients and also promote the use of generic drugs. Practice settings may also have established guidelines for what medications to prescribe for specific problems.

In the practice setting, the APRN may be confronted with challenges to adopting the role of prescriber. In states with considerable limitations on autonomous practice, collaborating physicians may challenge an APRN who writes a prescription that differs from his/her preference. Collaborative agreements may specify that the physician has the ability to override an APRN's prescribing decision.

The shift from professional preference and tradition to evidence-based practice has been shown to be a key strategy for achieving quality patient care (Ackley, Ladwig, Swan, & Tucker, 2008; Jacoby, Crawford, Chaudhari, & Goldfarb, 2010). Improved models for prescribing that increase the effectiveness of care and reduce error and cost are emerging from the rational prescribing and evidence-based care movements. These models use clinical practice guidelines, electronic health records, exert more control over pharmaceutical marketing, and promote standards for formularies (Crigger & Holcomb, 2007; Pedersen, Schneider, & Scheckelhoff, 2008).

Commitment to these models is essential for APRNs, whatever their level of autonomy, to improve the quality and safety of health. Recently educated APRNs, steeped in careful attention to rational and evidence-based prescribing, may encounter situations with colleagues who may be unaware of the most current medication information. These situations often require assertiveness and communication skills that facilitate collegial sharing about continuously changing knowledge.

Authority and responsibility

Prescriptive authority for APRNs may be sponsored by legislators who have limited understanding of the clinical abilities of the APRN (Safriet, 2002). Prescriptive authority carries responsibilities, even in states where collaboration or supervision is required. APRNs are accountable to patients, colleagues, the profession, and society for their actions, decisions, and practice (Pellegrino & Thomasma, 1993). As with any aspect of practice, errors or negligence in prescribing may result in disciplinary or legal action.

With all of the factors that influence the transition of the APRN as a prescriber, one certainty exists. There will be a degree of uncertainty, and often anxiety, about prescribing. The transition from facilitator of care as an RN to manager of care and prescriber as an APRN can be viewed as a professionally invigorating challenge or as a distressing situation.

Professional relationships

Implementation of the APRN role requires the development of strong relationships with other healthcare professionals, patients, the profession, and society. The time and effort needed to establish and maintain these relationships may be demanding. One study of NPs employed by United Healthcare EverCare indicated that 46% of the time that was designated as indirect care was spent communicating with other healthcare team members (Abdallah, 2005).

The transition from the RN to the APRN role may change APRNs' relationships with patients less than it changes their relationships with other healthcare professionals. The most dramatic change for APRNs is likely to occur with physicians. APRNs' level of prescribing expertise and the legal requirements of the prescriptive authority will influence their relationships with physicians. A physician may be a colleague in the true sense of the word or may serve as a consultant or supervisor. The relationship between an APRN and a physician at its best will be fulfilling, supportive, and truly collaborative with the interests of the patient at its core. A problematic relationship with a collaborating or supervising physician can serve as a barrier to APRN autonomy and compromise patient care. Furthermore, APRNs may experience isolation, invalidation, and marginalization (Kaplan & Brown, 2004; Martin & Hutchinson, 1999).

It is essential for APRNs to enhance their skills to manage and improve contentious professional relationships. APRNs who skillfully challenge and improve strained collegial relationships can build professional acceptance for all APRNs as well as enhance the quality of their own work life. These are situations where support and collaboration from other APRNs may be particularly effective. Some practices, however, may employ only one APRN, and time for collegial interaction at one's workplace may be limited.

The practice relationships that are legally required between APRNs and physicians vary from state to state. The majority of states still require some type of collaborative practice and some limit prescribing for specific medications or controlled drugs. For example, Alabama has the most restrictive scope of advanced practice in the United States and prescribing limits. These include:

- The drug type, dosage, quantity prescribed, and number of refills shall be authorized and signed by the collaborating physician;
- The drug shall be on the formulary recommended by the joint committee and adopted by the State Board of Medical Examiners and the Board of Nursing; and
- A certified registered NP or a CNM may not initiate a call-in prescription in the name of the collaborating physician for any drug, whether legend or CS, which the certified registered NP

is not authorized to prescribe under the protocol with certain exceptions (Alabama State Board of Nursing, 1995).

In states with restrictive practice laws, APRNs may be subject to direct oversight of the collaborating physician regardless of their expertise. Alabama and Florida do not allow APRNs to prescribe any CSs. In contrast, other states like Washington have no restrictions on APRN prescribing or any other aspect of practice (Pearson, 2011).

Beyond the legal requirement for collaboration, physicians may view APRNs differently from how APRNs view themselves. Fletcher, Baker, Copeland, Reeves, and Lowery (2007) conducted a study in a midwestern Veterans Health Administration region to describe NPs' and physicians' perceptions of the NP role, the degree of collegiality between the NPs and physicians, and the extent to which NPs felt accepted. NPs viewed themselves as autonomous and used physician collaborators in a consultation role. Physicians viewed the NPs as "extenders" used to "free-up their time." In both groups, the relationship between the physician and NP were seen as collegial, and physicians were satisfied with NP practice contributions.

Another study in a Pacific Northwest academic medical center revealed that physicians were supportive of NPs, respected their expertise, and that working with them was a positive experience (Soine, Errico, Redmond, & Sprow, 2011). Increased confidence in APRNs, appreciation of the enhancement of care received by patients, and a clearer understanding of the APRN scope practice were found in physicians who were currently working with APRNs.

The majority of physicians, however, did not understand the NPs' legal scope of practice in the state and the nature of NP educational preparation. Ten questions assessed study participants' knowledge about NP practice. Seventy-three percent of the physicians did not know that a graduate degree and a national certification were required for licensure as an NP in Washington State. Less than half (40%) of the physicians understood that the Washington State Nurse Practice Act authorizes full autonomy for NPs. Many (40%) also misunderstood the medical center bylaws and indicated that APRN supervision by physicians was required. Almost all

(90%) were unclear about the licensure differences between NPs and PAs. However, the physicians were more informed about NP prescribing than other aspects of NP scope of practice. Fifty-two percent of the physicians were aware of the legal authority of NPs to prescribe CSs. Another 26% thought this was true but were not completely certain.

The study's authors who were practicing APRNs at the medical center discussed the key contributions of APRNs to the medical center.

> [The] NP role has been conceptualized to add a qualitatively different fund of nursing knowledge and skills to the collaborative patient care team. NPs function as neither an attending nor resident substitute. Instead, NPs provide continuity of patient centered care and are a stable source for communication about patient care and facilitate transitions of patients across settings. Additionally, on many services, NPs facilitate interprofessional education as they actively participate in teaching and supervising residents. (Soine et al., 2011, p. 9)

Relationships with pharmacists are particularly important for the APRN prescriber. The pharmacist is the expert on pharmacological agents, while the APRN applies knowledge of medications contextually to the patient situation, patient preferences, and expectations of best practice. Ideally, APRNs work with pharmacists as colleagues who have the same goal of appropriate and safe medication management and a commitment to quality patient care.

A patient's pharmacological management may involve collaboration with a specialized practitioner, for example, a physician or APRN who practices in endocrinology. Different collaborative approaches may be used.

- A patient consultation is made with the specialist for evaluation and development of a medication regimen. The regimen is then implemented and monitored by the APRN.
- A patient is referred to a specialist who assumes care for specific health needs of the patient. The APRN typically maintains the role as the coordinator of care.

It is essential, however, that patients with a variety of complex problems who receive care from multiple specialists each of whom prescribes medications for a specific condition, have coordinated care by the APRN. The APRN serves in a vital role to assure that the patient's treatment plans are coordinated and monitored for drug interactions.

Strategies for success as a prescriber

Changes in evidence-based practice, patient-centered outcomes research, and the introduction of new medications require regular review of patient medication regimens. A professional development plan will help the APRN utilize the most current evidence in medication management.

Participation in lifelong learning is the essence of a professional development plan. Different forms of lifelong learning may include collegial mentoring by another APRN, participation in professional organizations, informal networking with colleagues, peer review, and continuing education seminars or online training that focuses on current medication management approaches. For example, Take Care Clinic, a national retail NP-based clinic, has a formal method of using peer review for quality improvement. This review process assures that patient encounters are evaluated and feedback about the treatment plan from a colleague is provided to the APRN. Collegial exchange such as chart review by peers can be a particularly powerful method of honing one's prescribing expertise (Sheahan, Simpson, & Rayens, 2001).

Efficient time management hinges on the APRN's medication management expertise. One approach to enhance prescribing effectiveness is to develop a "personal formulary" of medications one typically prescribes from different drug classes or for specific health conditions. This personal formulary is developed through current evidence, experience, patient feedback and responses to medications, and financial considerations.

Besides the use of a personal formulary, the APRN may employ strategies for prescribing drugs that save time and reduce the incidence of errors in medication management. Prescriptions that are computer generated or electronically submitted are increasingly common and reduce dispensing errors (Moniz et al., 2011). Use of health information technology is promoted by the Medicare and Medicaid Electronic Health Record Incentive Program which was a part of the American Recovery and Reinvestment Act of 2009. Despite the transition from handwritten to computer-generated prescriptions, the need to communicate with pharmacists continues and will facilitate medication monitoring and prescriptions renewal.

In the interest of safety, it is recommended that patients use one pharmacy only. In situations when the APRN is concerned a patient is abusing medications, there are programs through private and public health plans that can mandate use of one pharmacy only. Use of one pharmacy reduces medication errors, drug interactions, and multiple prescriptions from multiple providers for the same medication, particularly scheduled drugs.

An example of a public program that can mandate one pharmacy only is the Washington State Medicaid program known as *Patient Review and Coordination* which addresses overall excess utilization of services including medication use. A Medicaid client may be referred to the program for a variety of reasons, including two or more of the following medication-related criteria.

In a *90-day* period:

- Filled prescriptions at four or more pharmacies
- Received 10 or more prescriptions
- Had prescriptions written by four or more prescribers.

In a *one-month* period:

- Received prescriptions for CSs from two or more different prescribers.

When a Medicaid client is enrolled in the program, the use of only one pharmacy can be required (Washington State Medicaid, 2010).

As noted above, the transition to the prescriber role is part of the overall transition to APRN practice. Novice prescribers may require more time to consult references, electronic medication guides, and clinical guidelines. The effort usually required for a novice prescriber to select the most appropriate medication and write prescriptions can be extensive. Because the development of expertise will take time and occurs over months and years, APRNs are encouraged to have realistic expectations of the time required to develop ease and competence and be patient and kind to themselves during this process.

"The nature of decision-making, interactions, and expectations between prescribers and patients when choosing prescription drugs is a dynamic, multifaceted process" (Schommer, Worley, Kjos, Pakhomov, & Schondelmeyer, 2009, p. 167). An analysis of how patients, prescribers, experts, and patient advocates view the prescription choice process was conducted by Schommer, et al. (2009). Within the process of prescription drug decision making, five overall factors were identified: information, relationship, patient variation, practitioner variation, and role expectations. The researchers noted that "decisions regarding the selection and use of prescription medications are made by multiple individuals, at multiple times, in multiple locations, under different contexts and viewpoints. The prescription choice process may be complicated further by various abilities, beliefs, and motivations held by those involved in the decisions" (p. 167).

BARRIERS TO TRANSITIONING TO THE PRESCRIBER ROLE

Some barriers may impede rather than facilitate role transition and the APRN's assumption of the prescriber role. Prescribing is the aspect of the APRN role most commonly constrained by legal requirements for physician collaboration or supervision. Kaplan and Brown (2004) studied barriers to Washington State APRNs providing CSs prior to obtaining CSs prescriptive authority. The most common barriers were physician concern about possible liability as a collaborator, a physician and NP choosing different drugs, and physician reluctance to prescribe drugs selected by the NP. The study by Fletcher et al. (2007) noted above revealed different perceptions between NPs and physicians of advanced nursing practice. For APRNs in states with required collaborative agreements or supervision for prescribing, thoughtful conversations with a physician colleague may reduce misconceptions and discord. Even in states with autonomous prescribing, physicians who employ APRNs may expect to have input into an APRN's prescribing decisions.

A FRAMEWORK FOR PRESCRIBING
Rational prescribing

Rational prescribing rests on knowledge of the patient, knowledge about the nature of the health problem, and treatment using evidence-based guidelines, standards of care, and strategies for promoting medication use. With this information, the APRN and the patient make a shared decision through consideration of the benefits and burdens in the patient's particular situation. Both need to be mindful of the APRN's responsibility to act in the best interest of the patient. There are four general elements to rational prescribing: knowledge of the patient, knowledge of the disease and standard management, patient education and shared decision making, and maintaining a trust relationship with a patient.

Knowledge of the patient

Proper prescribing of medications requires careful evaluation of the patient with consideration of the patient's history, medication history, and physical assessment. A complete medication history includes herbal and nonprescription medications, prescription medications, recreational drugs, and all drug reactions. This more comprehensive approach involves assessing allergic responses, drug interactions, and family genetic propensities.

One important but often forgotten area of assessment is the patient's ability to manage his or her own medications. Names of drugs and the purpose of each drug may pose challenges for many patients. Assessment of the patient's motivation, cognitive abilities and attitudes about medication management, self-care, readiness to learn, health literacy, occupation, and educational background is essential to avoid false assumptions about the patient's ability to follow the healthcare plan. For example, a provider may incorrectly assume that a patient who is a nurse does not require the same counseling as other patients about medication side effects. Some patients with chronic problems may be more knowledgeable about their illness and medication management than the APRN. Others may be inexperienced, misinformed, and/or uninformed about the medications they use.

Knowledge of disease and standard management

APRNs continually gain experience and knowledge of the constantly changing area of pharmacological treatment. Rational prescribing is a method of drug management that is well established in international health and has become a cornerstone for prescribing medications. In 1985, the World Health Organization (2002) defined the rational use of medicines.

> Rational use of drugs requires that patients receive medications appropriate to their clinical needs, in doses that meet their own individual requirements for an adequate period of time, and the lowest cost to them and their community.

In addition to prescription medications, rational prescribing can include appropriate non-pharmaceutical management to supplement or replace drug therapy. The risk of polypharmacy, inappropriate treatment, and overtreatment are increased when rational prescribing is not used (Fulton & Allen, 2005; Van Vliet, Schuurmans, Grypdonck, & Duijnstee, 2006). Evidence-based practice guides rational prescribing and assures selection of appropriate drugs.

Little has been written in advanced nursing practice literature about rational prescribing, although outcomes related to irrational prescribing are well known (Crigger & Holcomb, 2007). Table 2.2 provides a summary of the four "rights" of rational prescribing. Box 2.1 is a set of recommendations to promote rational prescribing.

Concern for proper drug prescribing is not limited to the patient's individual needs but extends to the interests of different populations and the community. One way to reduce costs without compromising high-quality care is the use of generic drugs. Brand name drugs are usually prescribed for patients who have a strong preference, when generics fail or are not available. Safety of brand name drugs can also be an issue. When a medication is new to the market, there is less information about potential adverse consequences that may become apparent only after years of widespread use.

Some medications may not be appropriate for specific populations. The Beers criteria can be used to evaluate potentially inap-

Table 2.2 The four rational prescribing rights[a]

Any patient who receives treatment has a right to:
1. Appropriate medication for the need
2. Appropriate doses to meet individual requirements
3. Adequate clinical course
4. Lowest cost to patient and community

[a]Based on the World Health Organization definition of rational prescribing.

Box 2.1 Strategies for improving rational prescribing

- Resist prescribing for minor, self-limiting, or nonspecific symptoms.
- Avoid influences that can cloud rational decision making.
- Do not accept gifts that even have the *appearance* of affecting your decision making.
- Balance information received from the pharmaceutical industry with objective, unbiased sources.
- Encourage patients to seek out non-biased sources of information.
- Use evidence-based guidelines and electronic or current print references to assist in prescribing.
- Review patient medications during each visit.
- Emphasize lifestyle changes and always teach non-pharmacological management.
- Simplify and discontinue medications whenever possible.
- Avoid empirical treatment.
- Reduce the number of pharmacies and providers whenever possible.
- Titrate medication slowly.
- Monitor nonprescription drugs and treatments.

Source: Farrell, Hill, Hawkins, Newman, & Learned, 2003; Fick et al., 2003; Fulton & Allen, 2005; McVeigh, 2001.

---

propriate medications for adults 65 years or older. The criteria identify medications that should be avoided because they are ineffective, pose an unnecessarily high risk, or there is a safer alternative. The criteria also identify medications that should not be prescribed when the person has specific health problems (Farrell et al., 2003; Fick et al., 2003).

Many professional organizations publish clinical guidelines and standards of care that include strategies for prescribing. All APRNs, especially novice practitioners, benefit from these and other resources. A key aspect of rational prescribing is documentation of decisions. Refer to Chapter 8 for a full discussion of the importance of documentation.

Patient education and shared decision making
One of the greatest strengths of APRNs is the ability to develop a therapeutic relationship with patients and provide education

(Fletcher et al., 2007). APRNs also facilitate patient learning about pharmacological and non-pharmacological options. Shared decision making with the patient will result in an individualized plan of care that the patient is more likely to adopt. Emphasis on "knowing the patient" and exploring their attitudes about medication use helps practitioners avoid prescribing when the patient has no intention of taking a medication.

In the last decade, direct-to-consumer advertisement about medications has escalated with both positive and negative effects on patients (Crigger, Courter, Hamacher, Hayes, & Shepherd, 2009). Advertisements inform people about medications and symptoms related to certain disorders. Advertisements may also influence consumers to request unnecessary or inappropriate medications which makes rational prescribing more difficult. Studies of polypharmacy and direct-to-consumer advertising suggest some patients may request unnecessary medications that could be detrimental to their health (Ivanitskaya et al., 2010; Axtell-Thompson, 2005). APRNs, through education and counseling, can help patients understand these external influences and make an appropriate decision that reflects rational treatment choices.

Shared decision making should include a discussion of whether the use of medication is physically and financially sustainable, the accessibility of the treatment, and the ease of use. Patients should be informed of the most common and serious side effects as well as key monitoring tests that contribute to patient safety. For example, statins used to lower lipid levels may elevate liver enzymes or cause rhabdomyolysis. Patients should be informed of the rationale for periodic liver function testing and symptoms that could enable early detection if an untoward effect occurs. Many, however, have conducted considerable Internet research prior to their visit that in turn prompts medication questions or issues. Through education, a patient is provided relevant facts to make a decision about whether to take a medication. This is the process of informed consent (O'Keefe, 2001). Consent is typically verbal, but there may be situations in which written consent is obtained such as when using a medication off label. The phrase "off label" refers to when a medication is prescribed for a reason not approved by the Food and Drug Administration (FDA).

The APRN should not rely on the pharmacist as the sole educator about medications. The extent to which patients will actually read or understand a medication fact sheet provided by the pharmacist is unknown. Additionally, patients may read information about medications and become fearful of the potential side effects and not fill the prescription. APRNs may anticipate this situation by explaining it to the patient along with encouragement to return quickly for further discussion rather than discarding the prescription.

Novice prescribers are faced with developing a balance between providing too much or too little information about medications. Patients should be sufficiently informed to understand the action of a drug, the dosage, and the most common and severe adverse reactions. They also need to be informed about how to handle common problems, missing a dose, follow-up if the drug is not effective, and under what conditions the medication can be discontinued.

One last issue that may be overlooked is providing guidance about how long the patient should expect to take the medication. A guiding principle of prescribing is to use the lowest dose for the shortest period of time possible. An ideal medication is one that is effective with minimal or no side effects and is low cost. Sometimes, the patient's health issue resolves. Lifestyle modifications such as exercise and sodium reduction may result in lowered blood pressure. Weight loss in diabetics may improve the patient's glycemic levels. These may reduce or eliminate the need for medication.

Maintaining a trust relationship with the patient

APRN prescribing is based on choices about medications that reflect the patient's best interests. Decisions also reflect patient preferences. Additionally, the APRN should guard against participating in relationships that conflict with the patient's best interests. There is a substantial body of research that indicates gifts from the pharmaceutical industry, such as sponsored dinners, and pharmaceutical representative visits influence prescriber choices (Crigger, 2005; Crigger et al., 2009). Although voluntary rules are in place to limit the relationships and gifts, sample medications and educational programs continue to influence practitioners (see Chapter 6, The Influences of Pharmaceutical Marketing on APRN Prescribing).

Box 2.2 Strategies for working with patients

1. Educate the patient and provide written materials that substantiate your position. Ask the patient to do "homework" such as read specific websites or documents, listen to a program, and then return to discuss the treatment plan at a later time.
2. Always respect patients and listen to their comments. Active listening may validate their point of view and help them feel understood.
3. Respect the amount of time scheduled for the appointment while meeting the patient's need for discussion. Offer a follow-up appointment or use a telephone call or e-mail to continue the discussion.
4. Offer choices when possible to give the patient a sense of control and create a more positive encounter.
5. Provide information if a patient chooses to consult other providers.
6. Protect yourself. APRNs should never be bullied, subjected to abuse, or be threatened by physical harm. Consider *in advance* how you will handle a potentially threatening situation. Make a plan and share it with your colleagues. When in doubt, leave the room or have a colleague step into the room.

One of the most challenging aspects to prescribing can occur when patients have strong, erroneous, or unrealistic beliefs about their care. According to Grace (2009), some patients may be demanding, complaining, or rude, and require more extensive interaction than other patients. While these situations may prompt the label of "difficult patient," alternate terminology such as "difficult patient situations," "patients with difficult to treat situations," or "strong-willed" patients are more appropriate.

"Standing one's ground" with rational prescribing can be difficult in face of patients' demands for specific medications such as antibiotics. How can the APRN handle situations in which the patient assumes an adversarial role? Box 2.2 offers strategies to use when interacting with a patient who demands a certain type of treatment. Chapter 5, Managing Difficult Patient Situations, has a full discussion of this topic.

SPECIAL CONSIDERATIONS FOR PRESCRIBING
Overview

APRNs have clinical competencies to provide health care for diverse populations in diverse settings that may include emergency departments, primary care clinics, retail clinics, extended care facilities, prisons, and hospitals. Practice in these settings entails prescribing medications and other therapies and monitoring their effects.

New specialties have emerged based on the evolving healthcare environment and needs of the population. Examples of specialty areas that APRNs are selecting include, but are not limited to, oncology, geriatrics, dermatology, rheumatology, orthopedics, nephrology, cardiology, and palliative care. Within some of these specializations, pharmacological therapy often involves drugs and therapies not commonly used in the APRN's former setting, and there is often a need to acquire new knowledge. Additional needs and risks may be associated with prescribing in these specialized roles or in specialized settings. Adoption of the prescribing role will be influenced by factors such as the area of population focus or specialization, the setting, and the community.

Prescribing for specific populations

Many psychiatric mental health NPs work with children. There are few medications approved by the FDA for use with children with many mental health problems including depression, bipolar disorder, and schizophrenia. Conversely, there is an abundance of CSs marketed to treat children with attention deficit hyperactivity disorder (ADHD). This may lead parents to request these medications for behavioral issues even if the APRN does not diagnose ADHD.

The pediatric NP may prescribe medication for children from birth through 21 years of age and the family NP prescribes for children's concerns. Prescription challenges in this population sometimes involve calculating doses based on weight. As a vulnerable population, there is limited research on medication use in children. Consequently, a great deal of prescribing for children is not FDA approved and is known as "off label."

Geriatric NPs often work with patients who have polypharmacy complicated by mental and physical deficits. Polypharmacy increases the complexity of therapy, increases costs, and increases the risk of adverse consequences.

The types of drugs that CRNAs order and administer have potentially serious and immediate consequences. For example, when propofol is used for sedation, the CRNA must be alert to the rapid onset of action which is often within a minute. This rapid onset is dose-dependent and can result in an impaired respiratory drive, cause apnea, and require airway management.

CNMs, CNSs, and NPs must constantly consider the potential teratogenic effects of drugs in pregnant women. They must also consider the safety of drugs in lactating women. There are few randomized controlled trials regarding the safety of medications during pregnancy and lactation. To address this, the safety of medications is rated based on what information is available. Often the safety of a drug is unknown, and the APRN must proceed with caution.

NPs, CNSs, and CRNAs who work in pain management and palliative care typically prescribe a wide variety of CSs, often in large quantities. Pain management requires expertise both in selecting medications and in dealing with patients who request medications that may not be indicated. In contrast, APRNs who work with patients in palliative care may need to provide education to dispel concerns about addiction.

Other special considerations

An employer or health system may restrict APRN prescribing more than the law does. The VA is the largest employer of NPs nationwide. With over 6 million patients nationwide, VA patients often have a higher number of complex problems compared to the general public (Institute of Medicine, 2010). Polypharmacy and mental health issues among veterans who served in combat areas also pose a challenge (Fletcher et al., 2007).

Retail health clinics have proliferated during the last decade. These clinics limit what conditions the NP can manage, thus limiting what can be prescribed. Some specialty clinics such as family planning also use standardized protocols with a limited range of medication options.

There are many factors in the community that may pose the need for special prescribing considerations. These include the prevalence of various health problems and the degree of antibiotic resistance. The APRN may consider the prescribing preferences of his or her colleagues in a practice. Whether a health plan will cover a medication, the cost of medication, and whether a drug is on a retailer's reduced cost list are other special considerations when selecting drugs.

THE FUTURE OF THE APRN PRESCRIBING ROLE

Passage of the Patient Protection and Affordable Care Act (PPACA) in March 2010 created new opportunities for APRNs. When fully implemented, the PPACA will increase the number of people with healthcare insurance. There will be a pressing need for more healthcare providers, and APRNs are poised to fill this need. Prescribing may become more central to the APRN role as people who have had untreated problems for long periods of time enter the healthcare system. A balance between pharmacological and non-pharmacological treatment options may become more important as attention to cost-effectiveness and safety increases. The APRN has the opportunity to meet these demands using evidence-based practices and rational prescribing. As the evidence base for pharmacological treatments changes and the use of electronic prescribing increases, the APRN must adapt prescribing practices. Adoption of the prescriber role is a career-long process.

REFERENCES

Abdallah, L. M. (2005). EverCare nurse practitioner practice activities: Similarities and differences across five sites. *Journal of the American Academy of Nurse Practitioners, 17*(9), 355–362.

Ackley, B. J., Ladwig, G. B., Swan, B. A., & Tucker, S. J. (2008). *Evidence-based nursing care guidelines.* St.Louis, MO: Mosby.

Alabama State Board of Nursing. (1995). Nurse Practice Act Article 5, Advanced Practice Nursing §34-21-86. Retrieved from http://www.abn.state.al.us/UltimateEditorInclude/UserFiles/docs/admin-code/Chapter%20610-X-5.pdf

Arcangelo, V. P., & Peterson, A. M. (2006). *Pharmacotherapeutics for advanced practice: Practical approach* (2nd ed.). Philadelphia: Lippincott Williams & Wilkins.

Axtell-Thompson, L. M. (2005). Consumer directed health care: Ethical limits to choice and responsibility. *Journal of Medicine and Philosophy, 30*(2), 207–226.

Bauer, J. C. (2010). Nurse practitioners as an underutilized resource for health reform: Evidence-based demonstrations of cost-effectiveness. *Journal of the American Academy of Nurse Practitioners*, *22*(4), 228–231.

Brown, S. A., & Grimes, D. E. (1995). A meta-analysis of nurse practitioners and nurse midwives in primary care. *Nursing Research*, *44*(6), 332–339.

Brown, M. A., & Olshansky, E. (1998). Becoming a primary care nurse practitioner: Challenges of the initial year of practice. *Nurse Practitioner*, *23*(7), 46, 52–56, 58.

Brown-Benedict, D. J. (2008). The doctor of nursing practice degree: Lessons for the history of the professional doctorate in other health disciplines. *Journal of Nursing Education*, *47*(1), 448–457.

Brykcznski, K. A. (2009). Role development of the advanced practice nurse. In A. B. Hamric, J. A. Spross, & C. M. Hanson (Eds.), *Advanced practice nursing: An integrative approach* (4th ed., pp. 95–120). St. Louis, MO: Saunders Elsevier.

Congressional Budget Office. (1979). *Physician extenders: Their current and future role in medical care delivery*. Washington, DC: US Government Printing Office.

Crigger, N. J. (2005). Pharmaceutical promotions and conflict of interest in nurse practitioners' decision-making: The undiscovered country. *Journal of the American Academy of Nurse Practitioners*, *17*(6), 203–208.

Crigger, N. J., & Holcomb, L. (2007). Improving nurse practitioner practice through rational prescribing. *Journal for Nurse Practitioners*, *4*(2), 120–125.

Crigger, N., Courter, L., Hamacher, M., Hayes, K., & Shepherd, K. (2009). Public perceptions of healthcare participation in pharmaceutical marketing. *Nursing Ethics*, *16*(5), 647–658.

Deshefy-Longhi, T., Swartz, M. K., & Grey, M. (2008). Characterizing nurse practitioner practice by sampling patient encounters: An APRN study. *Journal of the American Academy of Nurse Practitioners*, *20*(5), 281–287.

Druss, B. G., Marcus, S. C., Olfson, M., Tanielian, T., & Pincus, A. (2003). Trends in care by nonphysician clinicians in the United States. *New England Journal of Medicine*, *348*(2), 130–137.

Dulisse, B., & Cromwell, J. (2010). No harm found when nurse anesthetists work without supervision by physicians. *Health Affairs*, *29*(8), 1469–1475.

Dunphy, L. M., Smith, N. K., & Youngkin, E. Q. (2009). Advanced practice nursing: Doing what had to be done – radicals, renegades, and rebels. In L. Joel (Ed.), *Advanced practice nursing* (pp. 2–22). Philadelphia: F.A. Davis.

Fairman, J. A., Rowe, J. W., Hassmiller, S., & Shalala, D. (2011). Broadening the scope of nursing practice. *New England Journal of Medicine, 364*(3), 193–196.

Farrell, V. M., Hill, V. L., Hawkins, J. B., Newman, L. M., & Learned, R. E., Jr. (2003). Clinic for identifying and addressing polypharmacy. *American Journal of Health-System Pharmacy, 60*(18), 1834–1835.

Fick, D. M., Cooper, J. W., Wade, W. E., Walter, J. L., Maclean, J. R., & Beers, M. H. (2003). Updating the Beers criteria for potentially inappropriate medication use in older adults: Results of a US consensus panel of experts. *Archives of Internal Medicine, 163*(22), 2716–2724.

Fletcher, C. E., Baker, S. J., Copeland, L. A., Reeves, P. J., & Lowery, J. C. (2007). Nurse practitioners' and physicians' views of NPs as providers of primary care to veterans. *Journal of Nursing Scholarship, 39*(4), 358–362.

Ford, J. (2008). 2008 in review: More growing pains. Twinges as the NP role expands. *Advance for Nurse Practitioners, 16*(12), 56–57.

Fulton, M. M., & Allen, E. R. (2005). Polypharmacy in the elderly: A literature review. *Journal of the American Academy of Nurse Practitioners, 17*(4), 123–132.

Grace, P. J. (2009). *Nursing ethics and professional responsibility in advanced practice*. Sudbury, MA: Jones & Bartlett.

Hamric, A. B., Spross, J. A., & Hanson, C. M. (Eds.). (2009). *Advanced practice nursing: An integrative approach* (4th ed.). St. Louis, MO: Saunders Elsevier.

Horrocks, S., Anderson, E., & Salisbury, C. (2002). Systematic review of whether nurse practitioners working in primary care can provide equivalent care to doctors. *British Medical Journal, 324*(7341), 819–823.

Institute of Medicine. (2010). *The future of nursing: Leading change, advancing health*. Washington, DC: The National Academies Press.

Ivanitskaya, L., Brookins-Fisher, J., O Boyle, I., Vibbert, D., Erofeev, D., & Fulton, L. (2010). Dirt cheap and without prescription: How susceptible are young consumers to purchasing drugs from rogue internet pharmacies? *Journal of Medical Internet Research*, *12*(2), E11.

Jacoby, R., Crawford, A. G., Chaudhari, P., & Goldfarb, N. I. (2010). Quality of care for 2 common pediatric conditions treated by convenient care providers. *American Journal of Medical Quality*, *26*, 1–6.

Kaplan, L., & Brown, M. A. (2004). Prescriptive authority and barriers to NP practice. *The Nurse Practitioner*, *29*(3), 28–35.

Kaplan, L., & Brown, M. A. (2006). What is "true" professional autonomy? *Nurse Practitioner*, *31*(3), 37.

Kaplan, L., Brown, M. A., & Simonson, D. C. (2011). CRNA prescribing practices: The Washington State experience. *AANA Journal*, *79*(1), 24–29.

Klein, T. (2008). Credentialing the nurse practitioner in your workplace: Evaluating scope for safe practice. *Nursing Administration Quarterly*, *32*(4), 273–276.

Laurant, M., Reeves, D., Hermens, R., Braspenning, J., Grol, R., & Sibald, B. (2009). Substitution of doctors by nurses in primary care. *Cochrane Database Systematic Reviews*, *1*. Retrieved from Cochrane Library database. doi: 10.1002/14651858.CD001271.pub2

Lenz, E. R., Mundinger, M. O., Kane, R. L., Hopkins, S. C., & Lin, S. X. (2004). Primary care outcomes in patients treated by nurse practitioners or physicians: two year follow up. *Medical Care Research and Review*, *51*(3), 332-351.

Lugo, N., O'Grady, E. T., Hodnicki, D. R., & Hanson, C. M. (2007). Ranking state NP regulation: Practice environment and consumer healthcare choice. *The American Journal of Nurse Practitioners*, *11*(4), 8–24.

Mantzoukas, S., & Watkinson, S. (2007). Review of advanced nursing practice: The international literature and developing generic features. *Journal of Clinical Nursing*, *16*(1), 28–37.

Martin, P. D., & Hutchinson, S. A. (1999). Nurse practitioners and the problem of discounting. *Journal of Advanced Nursing*, *29*(1), 9–17.

McVeigh, D. M. (2001). Polypharmacy in the older population: Recommendations for improved clinical practice. *Topics in Emergency Medicine*, *23*(3), 68–75.

Moniz, T. T., Seger, A. C., Klohane, C. A., Seger, D. L., Bates, D. W., & Rothschild, J. M. (2011). Addition of electronic prescription transmission to computerized prescriber order entry: Effect on dispensing errors in community pharmacies. *American Journal of Health-Systems Pharmacy*, *68*(2), 158–163.

National Council of State Boards of Nursing. (2010). Member board profiles. Retrieved from https://www.ncsbn.org/2010_Regulation_of_Advanced_Practice_Nursing.pdf

Newhouse, R. P., Stanik-Hutt, J., White, K. M., Johantgen, M., Bass, E., Zangaro, G., . . . Weiner, J. P. (2011). Advance practice nurse outcomes 1990–2008: A systematic review. *Nursing Economic$*, *29*(5), 1–22.

O'Keefe, M. E. (2001). *Nursing practice and the law*. Philadelphia: F.A. Davis Company.

Ohman-Strickland, P. A., Orzano, A. J., Hudson, S. V., Solberg, L. I., DiCiccio-Bloom, B., O'Malley, D., . . . Crabtree, S. F. (2008). Quality of diabetes care in family medicine practices: Influence of nurse practitioners and physician's assistants. *Annals of Family Medicine*, *6*(1), 14–22.

Pearson, L. J. (2011). The Pearson report. Retrieved from http://www.pearsonreport.com

Pedersen, C. A., Schneider, P. J., & Scheckelhoff, D. J. (2008). ASHP national survey of pharmacy practice in hospital settings: Prescribing and transcribing—2007. *American Journal of Health-System Pharmacy*, *65*(9), 827–843.

Pellegrino, E. D., & Thomasma, D. C. (1993). *The virtues in medical practice*. New York: Oxford University Press.

Phillips, S. J. (2007). A comprehensive look at the legislative issues affecting advanced nursing practice. *The Nurse Practitioner*, *32*(1), 14–17.

Prescott, P. A., & Driscoll, L. (1980). Evaluating nurse practitioner performance. *Nurse Practitioner*, *1*(1), 28–32.

Safriet, B. J. (1992). Health care dollars and regulatory sense: The role of advanced practice nursing. *Yale Journal on Regulation*, *9*(2), 417–488.

Safriet, B. J. (2002). Closing the gap between can and may in healthcare provider's scopes of practice: A primer for policymakers. *Yale Journal on Regulation*, *19*(2), 301–334.

Schommer, J. C., Worley, M. M., Kjos, A. L., Pakhomov, V. S., & Schondelmeyer, S. W. (2009). A thematic analysis for how patients, prescribers, experts, and patient advocates view the prescription choice process. *Research in Social and Administrative Pharmacy*, *5*(2), 154–169.

Schumacher, K. L., & Meleis, A. I. (1994). Transitions: A central concept in nursing. *Image: The Journal of Nursing Scholarship*, *26*(2), 119–127.

Sheahan, S. L., Simpson, C., & Rayens, M. K. (2001). Nurse practitioner peer review: Process and evaluation. *Journal of the American Academy of Nurse Practitioners*, *13*(3), 140–145.

Simonson, D. C., Ahern, M. M., & Hendryx, M. S. (2007). Anesthesia staffing and anesthetic complications during cesarean delivery: A retrospective analysis. *Nursing Research*, *56*(1), 9–17.

Soine, L., Errico, K., Redmond, C., & Sprow, S. (2011). Unpublished manuscript, under review.

Spitzer, W. O., Sackett, D. L., Sibley, J. C., Roberts, M., Gent, M., Kergin, D. J., . . . Olynich, A. (1974). The Burlington randomized trial of the nurse practitioner. *New England Journal of Medicine*, *290*(3), 252–256.

Ulrich, C. M., & Soeken, K. (2005). A path analytic model of ethical conflict in practice and autonomy in a sample of nurse practitioners. *Nursing Ethics*, *12*(3), 319–325.

Van Vliet, M. J., Schuurmans, M. J., Grypdonck, M. H., & Duijnstee, M. S. (2006). Improper intake of medication by elders—insights on contributing factors: A review of the literature. *Research & Theory for Nursing Practice*, *20*(1), 79–93.

Washington State Medicaid. (2010). Patient review and coordination program. Retrieved from http://hrsa.dshs.wa.gov/prr/index.htm

Weiland, S. A. (2008). Reflections on independence in nurse practitioner practice. *Journal of the American Academy of Nurse Practitioners*, *20*(7), 345–352.

World Health Organization. (2002). Promoting rational use of medicines: Core components. WHO Policy Perspectives on Medicines. Retrieved from http://whqlibdoc.who.int/hq/2002/WHO_EDM_2002.3.pdf.

Wright, W. L., Romboli, J. E., DiTulio, M. A., Wogen, J., & Belletti, D. A. (2011). Hypertension treatment and control within an independent nurse practitioner setting. *American Journal of Managed Care*, *17*(1), 58–65.

Creating a Practice Environment for Fully Autonomous Prescriptive Authority

3

Marie Annette Brown and Louise Kaplan

This chapter focuses on the range of external and internal barriers that can affect advanced practice registered nurses (APRNs) as prescribers. External factors are generally a part of the practice environment and include factors such as laws, regulations, policies, as well as the attitudes of other health professionals. Internal barriers are invisible or unacknowledged factors within the individual APRN, including personal characteristics such as conflict avoidance or the "need to be liked." Strategies to overcome internal and external prescribing barriers are offered as a way to generate enthusiasm among APRNs for facilitating change.

Chapters in this book highlight the multitude of opportunities and challenges advanced practice registered nurses (APRNs) confront when prescribing medications. Some opportunities and challenges result from laws, regulations, and policies that either promote or limit prescribing and are external to the individual. Other factors that are intrinsic to the individual, such as attitudes toward prescribing specific medications, may also promote or limit APRN prescribing.

The Advanced Practice Registered Nurse as a Prescriber, First Edition. Marie Annette Brown, Louise Kaplan.
© 2012 John Wiley & Sons, Ltd. Published 2012 by John Wiley & Sons, Ltd.

The external and internal factors described in this chapter are those that limit prescribing and serve as barriers. These barriers significantly restrict the potential for fully autonomous practice, the ultimate vision of APRNs.

Some APRNs work tirelessly to eliminate external and internal barriers to practice. Other APRNs do not perceive these barriers and accept restricted practice environments. Our research in Washington State suggests that "NPs in most states accepted physician control or supervision as a 'first step' in order to have any legal authorization to practice. Over the years, however, many NPs have accepted restrictions in autonomy which become normalized as 'good enough.' It may be easier for some NPs to maintain the status quo than to adopt a new scope of practice" (Kaplan & Brown, 2008b, p. 52). The fear that "making waves" could diminish job security and the cost of obtaining Drug Enforcement Administration (DEA) registration are common examples reported in our studies as deterrents to transitioning to more autonomous practice (Kaplan, Brown, Andrilla, & Hart, 2006). A core value that needs to be cultivated in APRN education and practice is commitment to actively work toward the goal of fully autonomous APRN practice nationwide.

Both external and internal barriers to prescribing medications are equally important to understand so that they can be addressed. Any prescribing barrier, no matter how small, affects the ability of APRNs to practice and provide comprehensive care to patients. Given the demands of practice in a complex healthcare system, it is critical to eliminate barriers to prescribing and attain the goal of creating a national practice environment for fully autonomous prescribing.

EXTERNAL BARRIERS
Federal laws and policies

Although states provide most regulation of prescriptive authority, the federal government affects certain aspects of prescribing. The most significant aspect is regulation of prescribing controlled substances (CSs). Any healthcare professional who prescribes Schedule II–V medications must register with the DEA or be working for a healthcare organization that has institutional DEA registration. Prescribing, dispensing, and administering scheduled drugs are regulated by the Controlled Substances Act of 1970 which can be accessed at http://www.justice.gov/dea/pubs/csa.html.

Some federal laws that restrict prescribing affect all healthcare professionals. For example, federal law requires that methadone, when used for opioid dependence, be administered or dispensed, but not prescribed, to patients only in licensed Opioid Treatment Programs (OTPs) (Food and Drugs, 2005). Federal law also stipulates "OTPs must ensure that opioid agonist treatment medications are administered or dispensed only by a practitioner licensed under the appropriate State law and registered under the appropriate State and Federal laws to administer or dispense opioid drugs, or by an agent of such a practitioner, supervised by and under the order of the licensed practitioner" (Public Health, 2003). These regulations do not prohibit a legally authorized provider from prescribing methadone for any condition other than addiction.

Another federal law excludes APRNs from prescribing Suboxone® (buprenorphine HCl/naloxone HCl dehydrate) and Subutex® (buprenorphine), which are indicated for treatment of opioid dependence. The Drug Addiction Treatment Act (2000) authorized only qualifying physicians to prescribe Suboxone and Subutex in the office-based setting.

Some federal laws that affect APRN prescribing are not always as obvious as those related to CSs. Medicare is the government-administered health plan for people aged 65 and older and some people with disabilities. Medicare requires that patients of certified home health agencies must be under the care of a physician although APRNs are often involved. All orders for home health patients, including medications, must be signed by a physician or the agency risks not receiving reimbursement from Medicare. Federal law does, however, allow an APRN to conduct a home visit to a home health patient, complete an evaluation, order medication and treatments, and bill for the visit (Buppert, 2009). An APRN may also provide office-based care to the home health patient and write prescriptions at that time.

State laws and rules that are prescribing barriers

All states authorize nurse practitioners (NPs) and certified nurse-midwives (CNMs) to prescribe, order, or furnish medications.

Some states, however, do not authorize clinical nurse specialists (CNSs) or certified registered nurse anesthetists (CRNAs) to prescribe. Only 34 states authorize CNSs to prescribe (National Council of State Boards of Nursing, 2010). Twenty-nine states authorize CRNAs to prescribe (Kaplan, Brown, & Simonson, 2011).

There are a variety of ways in which prescriptive authority is implemented for all APRNs and CRNAs serve an example. In two states and the District of Columbia, CRNAs are granted prescriptive authority as part of practice authority, and there is no physician involvement. Two states grant prescriptive authority with practice authority and require collaboration or supervision by a physician. Five states offer prescriptive authority separate from practice authority and without physician collaboration or supervision. Nineteen states grant CRNAs prescriptive authority separate from practice authority and *require* physician collaboration or supervision (Kaplan et al., 2011).

Even though all states authorize NPs to prescribe, order, or furnish medications, only 15 states and the District of Columbia (the number varies depending on the definition) have independent authority. Georgia and Illinois are among the states that allow prescribing only as a delegated authority. Georgia law is explicit that "ordering" a drug shall not be construed as prescribing. Box 3.1 is a section of the Georgia Board of Nursing rules authorizing prescriptive authority in Georgia. As a delegated act, the Georgia Medical Practice Act must also be referenced to have complete information about what is required for the APRN to order medications. Box 3.2 is one relevant section of the Georgia Medical Practice Act.

Illinois also has delegated prescribing authority. "A collaborating physician who delegates limited prescriptive authority to an advanced practice nurse shall include that delegation in the written collaborative agreement. The prescriptive authority may include prescription and dispensing of legend drugs and legend controlled substances categorized as Schedule III, IV, or V controlled substances, as defined in the Illinois Controlled Substances Act [720 ILCS 570] (Illinois Nursing and Advanced Practice Nursing Act, 2006)." Legislation passed in 2011 provides that a physician may (but is not required to) delegate authority to prescribe any Schedule II CS to an APRN if conditions are met.

Box 3.1 Georgia Board of Nursing selected rules on APRN prescriptive authority

(e) shall comply with the provisions of O.C.G.A. § 43-34-26.3 regarding prescription drug orders placed by an APRN for a drug or medical device including, but not limited to, the following:

1. no prescription drug orders submitted by an APRN for Schedule I or II controlled substances;
2. no refills of any drug for more than 12 months from the date of the original order, except in the case of oral contraceptives, hormone replacement therapy, or prenatal vitamins, which may be refilled for a period of 24 months;
3. no drug order or medical device that may result in the performance or occurrence of an abortion, including the administration, prescription or issuance of a drug order that is intended to cause an abortion to occur pharmacologically;
4. written prescription drug orders shall be signed by the APRN, be written on forms that comply with the nurse protocol agreement, and such forms shall contain the information required by paragraph (d) of O.C.G.A. §43-34-26.3;
5. a written provision in the nurse protocol agreement authorizing the APRN to request, receive, and sign for professional samples, and to distribute them to patients in accordance with a list of professional samples approved by the delegating physician that is maintained by the office or facility where the APRN works and that requires the documentation of each sample received and dispensed; and
6. compliance with applicable state and federal laws and regulations pertaining to the ordering, maintenance, and dispensing of drugs. (Georgia Registered Professional Nurse Act, 2007).

Box 3.2 Georgia Composite Board of Medicine rules on APRN prescriptive authority

(9) Provide that a patient who receives a prescription drug order for any controlled substance pursuant to a nurse protocol agreement shall be evaluated or examined by the delegating physician or other physician designated by the delegating physician pursuant to paragraph (2) of this subsection on at least a quarterly basis or at a more frequent interval as determined by the board.

Continued

(d) A written prescription drug order issued pursuant to this Code Section shall be signed by the advanced practice registered nurse and shall be on a form which shall include, without limitation, the names of the advanced practice registered nurse and delegating physician who are parties to the nurse protocol agreement, the patient's name and address, the drug or device ordered, directions with regard to the taking and dosage of the drug or use of the device, and the number of refills. A prescription drug order which is transmitted either electronically or via facsimile shall conform to the requirements set out in paragraphs (1) and (2) of subsection (c) of Code Section 26-4-80, respectively.

(e) An APRN may be authorized under a nurse protocol agreement to request, receive, and sign for professional samples and may distribute professional samples to patients (Georgia Composite Medical Board, 2009).

Qualified California NPs are issued a furnishing number to "order" or furnish drugs and devices according to approved standardized procedure or protocol. Prior to receiving a furnishing number, a certified NP must complete both an approved pharmacology course and a minimum of 520 hours of physician-supervised experience furnishing drugs and/or devices (California Business and Professions Code, 2004).

Some restrictions may seem minor, but when they exist in law, they must be followed and they limit full autonomy. In Utah, the law stipulates that an APRN who prescribes Schedule II and III CSs must do so in accordance with a consultation and referral plan (Utah Nurse Practice Act, 2009).

Beyond restrictions in prescribing are the additional limitations detailed in Chapter 7 that are related to dispensing medication samples, formularies, protocols, quantity limitation, co-signatures, mail-order medication prescription, and reciprocity in across-state prescribing. Georgia considers dispensing drug samples a delegated authority. In Illinois, the authority to receive and dispense samples must be part of the collaborative agreement. Alabama law requires physician collaboration in all aspects of prescribing with a written standard protocol. The protocol must "include a formulary of drugs, devices, medical treatments, tests and procedures that may be prescribed, ordered, and implemented by the certified registered nurse practitioner" (Alabama Nurse Practice Act, 2006). APRNs in Ohio who have a current, valid Certificate to Prescribe (CTP) must use a formulary developed by the Committee on Prescriptive Governance (Ohio Board of Nursing, 2009). The formulary designates medications that are approved for the holder of a CTP to prescribe and which medications may be prescribed only after a patient has been personally examined by the collaborating physician or the physician has authorized the prescription after consultation. The formulary also includes medications the APRN may not prescribe under any circumstances.

In states that require collaborative agreements or supervision for APRN prescribing, there are sometimes limits to the number of APRNs physicians can supervise. Alabama limits a physician to collaborate with or supervise no more than three full-time equivalent certified registered NPs, CNMs, and/or assistants to physicians. Florida also limits physician supervision in primary care to one principal practice location and no more than four satellite clinics, including specialty care, to the principal location and no more than two satellite offices (Pearson, 2011). This restricts the ability of APRNs to secure collaborating physicians, which has a ripple effect on prescribing.

Legal authorization to prescribe CSs is one of the underpinnings of fully autonomous practice. State law must authorize APRNs to prescribe CSs. At the time of this writing, only 15 states and the District of Columbia have laws that allow APRNs to prescribe CSs without direct physician involvement. As noted above, Utah requires a consultation and referral agreement to prescribe CSs II and III. Two states, Florida and Alabama, do not allow APRNs to prescribe CSs at all (Pearson, 2011). Six states allow CS prescribing for Schedule III–V drugs while other restrictions apply in some states.

Kentucky is an example of a state with many constraints on CS prescribing. CS II medications may be prescribed only for a 72-hour supply without refills. One of a few exceptions is for psychostimulants prescribed by psychiatric/mental health APRNs which may be for a 30-day supply. Schedule III prescriptions are limited to a 30-day supply while Schedule IV and V drugs may be prescribed with up to six refills (Kentucky Revised Statutes, 2010). There are other restrictions. Prescriptions for CS III combination hydrocodone products in liquid or solid dosage form are limited to a 14-day supply without refills. Diazepam (Valium®), clonazepam (Klonopin®), lorazepam (Ativan®), and alprazolam (Xanax®) prescriptions are also limited to a 14-day supply without refills. Carisprodol (Soma®) prescriptions are limited to a 30-day supply without refills (Kentucky Administrative Regulations, 2010).

Wisconsin APRNs also have restrictions related to CS prescribing. They may not prescribe, dispense, or administer any amphetamine, symphathomimetic amine, or compound designated as a Schedule II CS except as an adjunct to opioid analgesic compounds for the treatment of cancer-related pain, narcolepsy, hyperkinesis, drug-induced brain dysfunction, epilepsy, or depression refractory to other treatment and may not prescribe anabolic steroids to enhance athletic performance (Wisconsin Administrative Code, 2000).

In addition to the state laws and regulations that govern APRN prescribing, states sometimes have additional laws and rules that apply to all prescribers, especially related to CSs. While these are not specific to APRNs, the state laws still present another hurdle that can require time and effort, and cause confusion. For example, the federal Controlled Substances Act does not set an expiration date for a CS II prescription; however, states such as Washington have a 1-year expiration for all prescriptions while Oregon has a 2-year expiration. Some states require a special permit to prescribe CSs in addition to DEA registration. Connecticut requires that any practitioner authorized to prescribe, administer, and dispense controlled substances obtain a Connecticut Controlled Substance Registration prior to applying for DEA registration (Connecticut Department of Consumer Protection, 2009). In Ohio where APRNs require a collaborating physician, the medical board specifies conditions for which Schedule II stimulants may be prescribed. The conditions include narcoplepsy and behavior syndromes, such as attention deficit disorder. CS II stimulants may not be prescribed for weight reduction or control even if it is Food and Drug Administration approved (Ohio Administrative Code, 2009).

Problems also arise when states prohibit or restrict pharmacists from dispensing medication prescribed by APRNs from another state. In Kentucky and Texas, only prescriptions that conform to state law may be filled. For example, APRNs in Texas cannot write a prescription for a CS II drug. Consequently, a pharmacist cannot fill a CS II prescription from an APRN who is legally authorized to prescribe CS II drugs in his or her state (Pearson, 2011).

Marijuana is an illegal CS I drug, yet 13 states and the District of Columbia have medical marijuana laws. New Mexico and Washington are the two states that authorize NPs to be involved in the process. In order to stay within the confines of federal law that restricts prescribing marijuana, New Mexico NPs may refer qualified patients for medical marijuana. The state then grants permission to the patient (personal communication, J. Marshall, New Mexico Medical Cannabis Program; New Mexico Department of Health, 2009). The opportunity to recommend patients for medical marijuana may be of importance to APRNs who work in oncology, pain management, or with patients who have conditions such as multiple sclerosis or seizure disorders for which medical marijuana is indicated. The list of qualifying conditions will vary according to state.

Facility policies and limitations

A healthcare system, hospital, clinic, or private practice can develop policies that are more restrictive than state laws. These are usually developed by medical staff as part of the organization's bylaws. In a 2006 survey of Washington State CRNAs, some respondents reported that they experienced institutional barriers that prevented them from using prescriptive authority for scheduled drugs to provide anesthesia and analgesia care. These included hospital bylaws and malpractice insurance that did not cover CRNA prescribing (Kaplan et al., 2011). An example of a barrier to APRN practice that results from agency restrictions is one Veterans Administration (VA) facility that prohibits APRNs from prescribing CSs while other VA facilities in the state allow CS prescribing by APRNs. As one NP who requested anonymity communicated in an e-mail message:

> I work in the spinal cord injury clinic where a large number of our patients suffer chronic neuropathic pain. Not being able to prescribe pain medication for my patients has been a huge barrier to care. Occasionally there is no MD in the clinic and I must track down one on the inpatient unit . . . a huge inconvenience for both the patients and myself.

Even in states with autonomous prescribing, some individual providers, clinics, or agencies may have policies for prescribing that limit specific medications or categories of medications. Others may create policies that restrict APRN prescribing of specific medications or classes of drugs. One APRN reported that the medical director of an emergency department prohibited all providers from prescribing azithromycin "Z-packs." Another APRNs worked with a collaborating physician who barred APRNs from prescribing antidepressants for an unexplained reason. Also problematic is that organizations sometimes limit the kind of health issues an APRN may treat. For example, APRNs working in retail clinics are limited by corporate policy to provide care for specified common acute problems. This restriction limits prescribing. Take Care Clinic™ advertises that patients 18 months and older are treated for respiratory illnesses, skin conditions, minor injuries, diagnostic testing, wellness, vaccinations, physicals, and "additional treatments." Additional treatments refers to problems such as bladder infections, fever, head lice, otitis externa, and conjunctivitis (Take Care Clinic™, 2009).

Some prescribing limitations may occur when there is lack of familiarity with APRN background and expertise. For example, facilities or clinics have required APRNs to demonstrate competency beyond the state's educational requirements. The requirements include additional coursework in pharmacology or examinations about a specific body of prescribing knowledge.

Other barriers

Additional barriers can exist in the community, specifically related to pharmacies or pharmacists, their policies, and practices. A landmark case in Washington State involved a pharmacy that refused to fill prescriptions for Plan B contraception. The Washington State Board of Pharmacy subsequently issued rules requiring pharmacies and pharmacists to assure that a prescription was filled in a timely manner while allowing for an individual pharmacist to refuse to dispense a prescription. The refusal of any pharmacist to dispense a medication such as Plan B affects all prescribers, including APRNs and their patients. The pharmacy that refused to dispense Plan B filed suit against the Washington State Department of Health. An injunction exempted this pharmacy from complying with the rule until the suit was settled. All other Washington State pharmacies must comply with the rule (Americans United for Separation of Church and State, 2009). Kaplan and Brown (2004, 2006), and Sherman, Fuller, and Hunter (1999) identified issues pertaining to pharmacists' refusal to accept telephone prescriptions from APRNs. Some APRNs report difficulty having prescriptions filled by a mail-order pharmacy (Pearson, 2011).

Organized medicine has a deep philosophical commitment to physician supervision of APRNs despite decades of research that confirm APRNs provide safe, quality care (Brown & Grimes, 1995; Congressional Budget Office, 1979; Dulisse & Cromwell, 2010; Horrocks, Anderson, & Salisbury, 2002; Laurant et al., 2006; Lenz, Mundinger, Kane, Hopkins, 2002; Lenz, Mundinger, Kane, Hopkins, & Lin, 2004; Newhouse et al., 2011; Ohman-Strickland et al., 2008; Prescott & Driscoll, 1980; Safriet, 1992; Simonson, Ahern, & Hendryx, 2007; Spitzer et al., 1974). The AMA scope of practice monograph on NPs reflects this stance on supervision of APRNs (American Medical Association, 2009). Despite opposition to APRN prescribing and autonomous practice on the local, state, and federal levels, it is imperative to emphasize many physicians have collegial and supportive relationships with APRNs. As an example, Washington State organized medicine lobbied vigorously for a Joint Practice Agreement (JPA) with a physician as part of compromise legislation to allow APRNs to prescribe CSs II–IV. When the JPA requirement was implemented, the majority (81%) of Washington State APRNs responding to a statewide survey noted that their collaborating physician was not involved in their daily prescribing practice and that the JPA was, for the most part, a formality with no restrictions. Some APRNs' (16%) only contact with the physician was to set up the JPA (Kaplan, Brown, & Donahue, 2010).

Barriers in states with required physician involvement
In states that require physician involvement in prescribing (e.g., supervision, collaborative agreements, protocols), barriers exist that may discourage APRN prescribing or limit patient access to necessary medications. Physicians may be reluctant to enter into collaborative agreements or provide supervision because of concerns about increased liability. Prior to obtaining prescriptive

authority for CSs II–IV in Washington State, APRNs reported that physician concern about vicarious liability was the most common barrier to providing prescriptions for CSs (Kaplan & Brown, 2004). Vicarious liability is legal liability based on a relationship rather than on actions. It occurs when a relationship exists between A and B, such that courts will impose liability upon A if, through negligence, B injures C to whom B has a responsibility for care (Jenkins, 1994). Generally, malpractice liability and insurance premiums do not increase when a physician enters a collaborative relationship with an NP (Buppert, 2003).

Competition with other providers, negative attitudes about APRNs, or preference for collaboration with physician assistants (PAs) may limit physician willingness to collaborate with or supervise APRNs where it is required by law. Also, there may be monitoring of prescriptions and/or detailed record keeping required of the APRN.

Certain laws make the logistics of prescribing a challenge. In Michigan, prescriptive authority for a Schedule II drug cannot be delegated unless the APRN is employed by a hospital, freestanding surgical outpatient facility, or hospice (Michigan Nurses Association, 2009). In any other setting, a physician's signature is required for a Schedule II prescription. This creates an access to care problem when the physician is not immediately available.

Protocols for prescribing may limit both the number and type of medications necessary for comprehensive practice and require APRNs to select medications based on their physician colleagues' preferences. This constrains the APRN's ability for evidence-based rational prescribing and decision making based on in-depth knowledge of the patient. In states where APRNs are authorized to prescribe scheduled drugs only if they are included in a protocol, a physician collaborator may be unwilling to authorize this type of prescribing. Furthermore, the physician may select a different drug than the one requested by the APRN. When required to refer patients to physicians for certain medications, there is a possibility that the patient may transfer care to the physician.

Challenges accessing complete and accurate information

It is essential for APRNs to be knowledgeable about and practice in accordance with state and federal laws. Locating and understanding scope of practice information may be challenging. Some websites for boards of nursing do not clearly indicate where to find information or the information is not available or updated. This information may be available only by telephone contact with a staff person. The level of familiarity among state board staff with APRN scope of practice issues will vary. Only a few boards have a specific person dedicated to address APRN issues.

There are many interesting examples of the challenges noted above. In 2009, a law in Vermont eliminated the formulary requirement for APRNs. The Board of Nursing deleted the link to the formulary from its website; however, statements indicating the requirement to use a formulary were inadvertently left on the website for many months. The Georgia Board of Nursing website contains many of the rules for APRN prescribing. However, because prescribing is a delegated authority and the remainder of the rules are on the Board of Medicine website, APRNs may not realize the necessity to review both sets of rules.

In Michigan, prescriptive authority is also a delegated act but is not based on a law as is the case in most states. Instead, prescriptive authority is based on an Attorney General opinion that a 1978 law allowing physicians to delegate prescribing to a physician's assistant also allowed delegation of prescribing to a licensed professional nurse. The Michigan Nurses Association has a section of its website dedicated to explaining advanced practice and prescriptive authority. This is a major contribution as there is limited information available through the Board of Nursing. This information may be accessed at http://www.minurses.org/apn/apn-npfaq.shtml.

There are alternate sources of information that reduce barriers for APRNs. These include scope of practice information available from local, state, and national nursing and APRN organizations and journals and their respective websites. Information about prescribing CSs in accordance with federal law can be obtained through the DEA at http://www.justice.gov/dea/index.htm. APRNs authorized to prescribe CSs need to determine whether there are additional state-specific requirements.

INTERNAL BARRIERS TO PRESCRIBING

Internal barriers are often invisible or unacknowledged factors within the individual APRN and can be overlooked when analyzing barriers to APRN prescribing. For example, lack of expertise to prescribe a specific medication or class of medications and the time required to obtain this information *are* internal barriers. For CSs, internal barriers may include aversion to patients perceived to have drug-seeking behaviors and/or the responsibility of prescribing CSs.

Internal barriers may arise when APRN education does not include the full range of prescribing competencies. Role socialization may also contribute to the development of internal barriers. Professional attitudes and values are developed through the educational environment, interactions with other healthcare professionals, and community practice norms. These attitudes and values shape an individual's approach to prescribing and contribute to the development of a full range of prescribing competencies.

Prescribing competencies must include the ability to effectively communicate with patients in challenging clinical situations. Patients may request specific medications such as antibiotics, CSs, or brand name drugs they identify from direct-to-consumer advertising (see Chapter 6). APRNs may have a variety of reactions to these requests ranging from resistance to acquiescence to acceptance (see Chapter 5). Skillful APRN prescribers can help patients and families understand what types of medications are and are not appropriate for particular situations. An exemplar of national efforts to assist all prescribers with these challenges is the Centers for Disease Control and Prevention's program using evidence-based guidelines to promote judicious antibiotic prescribing. "Get Smart: Know When Antibiotics Work" has resources for the public and healthcare professionals and can be accessed at http://www.cdc.gov/getsmart/.

Another issue, resistance to prescribing CSs, may stem from the APRN's perception that the patient is exhibiting "drug-seeking behavior." Requests for widely advertised, brand-name drugs are common. Information alone about the equivalency of generic and brand-name drugs and the cost differential may not change patient preferences. Prescribing decisions are ideally made based on a patient-centered approach and "knowing the patient" to tailor the discussion in light of the patient's decision-making approaches. These situations emphasize the importance of skills such as APRN assertiveness and negotiation.

Internal barriers can also arise from an individual APRN's biases about a drug category, such as CSs or weight-loss medications. Self-reflection about the source of the bias is essential to assess the extent to which a decision is evidence based. Individual biases that serve as internal barriers may also be influenced by colleagues in the larger professional community.

Chronic noncancer pain is a common reason patients seek health care and is often inadequately treated. As part of an effort to address this problem, the U.S. Congress declared the "Decade of Pain Control and Research" beginning in 2001. The Joint Commission, an accrediting agency, issued pain management standards in 2000 that support the right of individuals to appropriate pain management (American Pain Society & American Academy of Pain Medicine, 2009).

Prescribing CSs may evoke a constellation of concerns that prompt some APRNs to avoid the responsibilities associated with these drugs. These concerns include issues such as the potential for patient addiction or diversion. APRNs may fear legal or disciplinary action despite data that these risks are very low.

To investigate the substance of the fear of disciplinary action when prescribing CSs, information about disciplinary cases by the Washington State Nursing Care Quality Assurance Commission against APRNs between August 2001 and March 2007 was reviewed. No action was taken against an APRN for overprescribing or underprescribing CSs. Only six cases resulted in action related to CSs of which three involved diversion for personal, nontherapeutic use and four involved prescribing without prescriptive authority for CSs (Kaplan & Brown, 2008a).

Subsequent to this review, one APRN had her licensed suspended in 2007 for inappropriately prescribing narcotics for two patients who were known substance abusers. The patients had also received opioids from other providers. Another APRN was disciplined in 2010 for prescribing extremely high doses of opioids to patients without appropriate assessment or ongoing monitoring. This represents a low risk of disciplinary action in a state with over 4000 APRNs. Nonetheless, some APRNs may choose to develop a practice that excludes providing care for patients who require CSs.

Development of prescribing competencies through appropriate education and training provides the essential foundation for practice. The early decades of NP role development provided few opportunities for identifying and implementing prescribing competencies. The current healthcare environment presents daunting challenges from the overwhelming amount of information necessary for competent prescribing.

Lack of knowledge about a specific drug or class of medications is an internal barrier that may limit an APRN's ability to provide comprehensive care. APRNs may describe this situation by stating they have "no need" for specific medications or that they are not comfortable or competent in a specific area of prescribing.

At the same time, it is essential that APRNs prescribe within the scope of their practice and their knowledge base. Self-assessment of limitations is central to safe, quality practice. It is also important to emphasize that providers are not responsible for prescribing every class of medication. Professional autonomy provides the foundation for each APRN to create an individualized approach to safe, quality practice.

Another important aspect of internal barriers relates to the APRN's sense of autonomy. State laws, community standards, and practice policies may lead to a limited perspective among some APRNs and other health professionals about APRN autonomous prescribing. Over time, norms often develop that perpetuate acceptance of these restrictions. In Washington State, which has independent practice authorized since 1973 and fully autonomous complete prescriptive authority since 2005, only 83% of respondents to an APRN survey reported that they felt fully autonomous (Kaplan et al., 2010). Ambivalence about autonomous practice and prescribing as well as the willingness to accept practice limitations serve as internal barriers to autonomous prescribing.

STRATEGIES TO ADDRESS PRESCRIBING BARRIERS

The elimination of both external and internal barriers is vitally important to attain fully autonomous prescribing nationwide. Change requires proactive strategies on multiple levels. Strategies to promote fully autonomous prescribing include a range of actions from individual self-assessment and reflection to lobbying for changes to state or federal law.

Development and implementation of these strategies requires consideration of the sociocultural context and prescribing environments which vary widely across the nation. For example, cultural norms and gender politics about women's access to power and self-determination may be more limited in some communities. Consequently, APRNs may utilize different approaches to change in different states.

The elimination of both external and internal barriers is essential. Legislative activities, regulatory change, and advocacy contribute to the elimination of external prescribing barriers. Little attention, however, has been paid to internal barriers. Some APRNs may normalize a supervised or constrained environment or report "no need" to expand their scope of practice. An individual or small group of APRNs with a broader view can "raise the consciousness" of their practice colleagues and champion changes in their individual setting. Often, a key first step is bringing together the APRNs in a practice or organization to obtain a fuller picture of the constrained APRN practice environment. A deeper understanding of the advantages of "what might be possible" can strengthen APRNs' commitment to change. Local, state, and national professional groups and organizations can be a source of evidence-based, well-designed literature advocating the benefits of fully autonomous APRN practice to patients and the healthcare systems. It is also essential for APRN faculty to prepare the next generation of APRNs with the expectation of autonomy. Faculty can strengthen curriculum that develops students' skills and commitment to initiate change in the complacency that may exist in their new practice environment. New graduates who understand their responsibility to changing their immediate practice environment can inspire colleagues with their enthusiasm. Faculty and student commitment to this vision can help build expertise in implementation of strategies to facilitate readiness for change to fully autonomous APRN practice and prescribing.

ELIMINATING EXTERNAL BARRIERS TO PRESCRIBING
Legislative activities
While most prescribing is regulated by the states, federal laws and rules may impinge on APRN prescribing. Organized, complex, and multifaceted approaches are required to make federal level changes in health policy. Over the decades, APRN and nursing organizations have recognized the need for consensus regarding

proposed policy changes as well as the necessity to have a coordinated lobbying effort. It literally "takes an act of Congress" to change and/or create laws that promote APRN practice and prescribing.

The Nurse Practice Act (NPA) generally defines APRN scope of practice although several states involve the Board of Medicine or other entities. The NPA is created by legislators who often lack an understanding of APRN expertise. Consequently, it is important to develop a cadre of politically competent APRNs who can serve as consultants to policymakers and their staff (O'Grady & Johnson, 2009). Relationships with legislators provide the foundation to encourage them to become sponsors and champions of bills that improve APRN scope of practice, including autonomous prescribing. Success in passing APRN legislation may require years of lobbying to educate legislators and gain their support. Effective lobbying results from strong nursing organizations and creation of coalitions among APRNs. As APRN and public interests are usually carefully aligned, it is important for APRNs to participate in public discourse on health policy issues. APRNs can utilize their expertise to support legislation that promotes access to care, reduction of health disparities, and enhances quality of patient care (O'Grady & Johnson, 2009). Box 3.3 recommends education of policymakers about the benefits of APRN practice and highlights information necessary for this process. Box 3.4 provides an overview of the key elements involved in lobbying for legislative changes.

Successful interactions in the policy arena require effective communication. Underlying principles for communication include:

- Use clear, thoughtful language that avoids jargon and presents one's expertise.
- Accurate, evidence-based information establishes credibility.
- Describe a problem without complaint and provide a realistic solution.
- Articulate how an issue has relevance beyond nursing.
- Use examples from professional practice to move an issue from the abstract to the concrete and "make it real."
- Avoid the use of language that is sarcastic, demeaning, and inflammatory even if confronted by proposals or positions that

---

Box 3.3 Recommendation: educate policymakers about the benefits of NP practice

While NPs are educated to provide comprehensive care, legal and policy restrictions continue to limit their practice. As the population ages and healthcare problems become increasingly complex, restrictive practice environments lead to the underutilization of NP skills, knowledge, and abilities. Ultimately, policymakers need to formulate laws and regulations that result in autonomous practice to improve access to evidenced-based quality patient care provided by NPs. Information needed to educate policymakers on the importance of fully autonomous NP practice includes:

- The skills, knowledge, and abilities of NPs
- Databased analyses of the outcomes of NP care
- The influence of autonomy on NP practice and access to patient care.

  In addition, NPs should:
- Secure adequate funding for additional research about the quality and safety of NP care
- Evaluate the "cost" of restrictions on NP practice to the patient, the insurer, and society.

Box 3.4 Influencing legislative change

To effect change in your state's legislature, consider basic steps compiled from the state of Washington's website:

Know how the process works
Consult your state government's website for an overview of the legislative process and contact information for legislators.

Make yourself the expert
Do your homework: know who the issue affects, what others feel about it, how it will influence future trends, and any other important contextual information to the issue at hand. Combining this with your own personal experience is the most effective information you can provide.

Get to know your legislators
You can contact your legislators in a number of ways:

- Personal visit. Call the office, introduce yourself, tell the legislator or the legislative assistant what you would like to discuss, and make an

Continued

57

appointment for a visit. Use the Member Rosters to find the phone numbers. If you plan a visit, be prepared for your discussion. Know what you want to say, be factual, and make your comments as brief and specific as you can.

- Attend a Town Hall Meeting. Most legislators conduct periodic town hall meetings at various locations in their district.
- Write a letter or e-mail. Make your message to the point, clear, and formal. Include your full contact information so the legislator can respond via email or letter. Use the Member Rosters to find contact information for specific legislators.
- Testify before a committee. Be prepared to articulate your views and positions at a public hearing on an issue or bill.

Get to know legislative staff
Legislators rely heavily on professional staff for information gathering and analysis. They work on a wide range of issues and always appreciate new sources of clear and accurate information. Members of the staff can also supply you with the most current information available.

Network with other citizens
Find out whether there are groups that share your concerns and establish a network. A group of concerned citizens can be much more effective working together, rather than as separate individuals trying to accomplish the same goal.

Source: Adapted from Washington State Legislature. *A Citizen's Guide to Effective Legislative Participation*. Retrieved April 4, 2011, from http://www.leg.wa.gov/legislature/Pages/EffectiveParticipation.aspx

are inaccurate, debasing, or that diminish the contributions of APRNs.

Regulatory changes
Regulatory change involves development of rules that may be necessary to implement a law as well as to fulfill the legislative mandates of governmental agencies. For example, a state's law that authorizes prescriptive authority with physician involvement requires rules to specify the precise nature of that involvement.

States have administrative procedures acts that delineate the legal process for creating rules and afford the opportunity for public participation. It is imperative that APRNs participate in the regulatory process which is equally important as passing laws. Often, "the devil is in the detail," and the rules and implementation directly affect each APRN's practice experience.

APRNs individually or through professional organizations need to insure that they are apprised of proposed rules that need to be analyzed to determine their impact on APRN practice. Comments can be sent in writing or given as testimony at a hearing. For example, rules may be proposed in a state to require physician-supervised practice hours to qualify for autonomous prescribing. APRNs could oppose this rule by providing APRN prescribing competencies developed in educational programs and evidence from other states with fully autonomous prescribing.

Advocacy

Advocacy involves active support for a cause or position. Advocacy about the APRN role and competencies most often occurs during daily interactions with patients and colleagues. The need for advocacy, however, extends to a multitude of issues from those in the workplace to national health policies. A great deal of advocacy occurs during the legislative and regulatory process. Advocacy also includes activities such as responding to misrepresentations of NP practice by the American Medical Association; raising public awareness through media campaigns; community service to promote the APRN role; and participation in health-related and community advisory boards. Advocacy often occurs on an individual level, for example, sending a letter to the editor of a media outlet that publishes or reports an inaccurate or limited view of APRN practice. Advocacy can be direct or indirect. Membership in national APRN organizations supports their efforts to be a strong voice for APRNs on issues such as assuring provider neutral language in health policies.

Prescribing-related advocacy provides an opportunity for APRNs to contribute to health policy at multiple levels. APRNs can challenge pharmaceutical companies to change package labeling and marketing materials to use the term healthcare provider rather than doctor. APRNs practicing at a state psychiatric facility, for example, may need to advocate for changes in or exceptions to the state drug formulary that prevents them from providing a specific antipsychotic medication proven effective for a specific patient.

Community-level advocacy is clearly needed to change small but significant perpetuation of APRN invisibility. For example, most automated messages used by pharmacies refer to doctors or doctors' representatives and need to be replaced by inclusive language of prescribers or providers. This situation provides important opportunities for reminding pharmacy management and business owners about the widespread contribution of APRN prescribers.

APRNs who educate their colleagues and supervisors about their legal scope of practice can advocate for the elimination of prescribing barriers that arise at a facility or in a practice. Facility or practice level APRN councils, even when a small number of APRNs are involved, can lend credibility to advocacy efforts. Individuals are urged to assure that collaborative agreements do not include requirements beyond what the law stipulates.

Developing political competence for effective advocacy

APRNs will be most successful in their efforts to achieve fully autonomous prescribing when they achieve political competence in their interprofessional interactions. It is critical for APRNs to maintain their integrity and professional approach while being passionate but considered as they advocate for change. When APRNs develop consensus and cohesion, they promote an environment in which they are respected, trusted, and effective. O'Grady and Johnson (2009) eloquently articulate this perspective in their discourse on "Using Force versus Power" (see Box 3.5).

Learning practical skills to influence policy positions the APRN to be effective in a variety of professional arenas. Many APRNs already have these skills honed from their professional experience and/or develop them further during graduate education. To enhance expertise, APRNs can attend educational offerings focused on policy. A mentor or experienced colleague can guide novices in the policy process. Volunteering for a professional organization's legislative or political action committee is an opportunity to gain direct experience and develop skills.

Box 3.5 Barriers to political competence

Using force versus power

Power accomplishes with ease what force, even with extreme effort, cannot. On the interpersonal front, it is important for APRNs to avoid using force in advancing their positions in the policy arena. This is commonly done by nurses participating in interdisciplinary policy or problem-solving meetings. The twin approaches of being judgmental and parochial can quickly compromise effectiveness. *Judgmentalism*, or criticizing other people or disciplines, distracts from effective problem solving and in the process can reflect poorly on the judger, taking away the power to influence. When we diminish others or the work they do, we can provoke defensiveness and consequently limit ourselves and our capacity to influence others meaningfully. *Nursing parochialism* occurs when nurses present a narrow, restricted scope or outlook in which only nursing and nursing's interests are offered as solutions. These postures in the policy arena (or any other setting) do not build wide-based support or strong relationships. APRNs' potential impact on cost, quality, and access, if fully unleashed, is a powerful solution to some of the most perennial healthcare problems of our time. Power is characterized by humility and truth, which needs no defense or rhetoric—it is self-evident. Force is divisive and exploits people for individual or personal gain (Hawkins, 2002). For APRNs to be effective in influencing policy, a great degree of maturity, discipline, restraint, and respect for self and others must be practiced.

Source: Reprinted from O'Grady and Johnson (2009), with permission from Elsevier Publishing Ltd.

APRNs need to be prepared for changes in scope of practice. Education and outreach that informs APRNs, policymakers, and other health professionals of impending changes can facilitate adoption of new laws and regulations. Box 3.6 identifies a variety of strategies that can be used.

ELIMINATING INTERNAL BARRIERS TO PRESCRIBING

As APRNs engage in activities to eliminate external barriers and pass legislation that enables fully autonomous prescribing, attention to the elimination of internal barriers is equally as important. Moreover, efforts to prevent internal prescribing barriers need to

---

Box 3.6 Recommendation: prepare NPs for a new scope of practice before legislation actually passes

Readiness for change could be enhanced by efforts to transition NPs to a new scope of practice prior to the passage of legislation. Possible strategies to transition NPs to a new scope of practice include the following:

- Develop a plan to prepare NPs for scope of practice changes.
- Include formal and informal discussions at NP conferences and meetings.
- Send informational mailings about the rationale for pending legislation to all NPs licensed within a state (may require special funding).
- Encourage healthcare organizations that employ large numbers of NPs to disseminate information using their internal communication mechanisms.
- Work with the media to communicate ongoing legislative activities.
- Work with legislators to include NP legislative activities in their newsletters.
- Develop a collaborative project among all NP groups and professional organizations within the state to establish a website dedicated to the implications of impending legislation.

---

begin in APRN educational programs. When internal barriers develop, they are often unacknowledged and can be more difficult to address than external barriers.

Role development in APRN programs

One component of APRN education is facilitating the transition of students from the role of administering medication to the role of prescribing medication. Course content and its application in clinical situations serve as the foundation for the prescriber role. APRN students develop prescribing competencies and expertise relevant to their scope of practice.

Some APRN educational programs are located in states that restrict APRN prescribing, particularly for CSs. Nonetheless, APRN programs are responsible for unambiguous socialization of students to assume the responsibilities of prescribing, including CSs. This is critical because complete prescriptive authority is an essential component of fully autonomous practice. It is also important to prepare future APRNs in these states for scope of practice changes. APRN prescribing education that is consistent across states enhances professional mobility and prepares APRNs to practice in any state.

Professional development for the experienced APRN

APRNs who prescribe in restrictive environments are prone to developing internal barriers because they lack opportunities to utilize a full range of prescribing competencies. People tend to adapt to these environments and become less aware of their impact. Continuing education, conferences, journals, professional associations, and mentors are mechanisms to enhance awareness of these restrictions and encourage APRNs to overcome internal barriers.

Continuing education (CE) sessions typically update knowledge and prescribing competencies. CE can also address internal barriers and develop skills needed to deal with difficult situations, such as unwarranted requests for CSs. Professional conferences and meetings can serve as forums for APRNs to discuss internal barriers to prescribing and develop strategies to overcome them. APRN journals provide evidence-based prescribing information that supports a full scope of autonomous prescribing.

Another common internal prescribing barrier is fear of disciplinary action, particularly about prescribing CSs. An experienced colleague or mentor can provide guidance and foster confidence.

IMPLICATIONS

External and internal prescribing barriers limit the ability of APRNs to reach their full professional potential. APRNs who practice in restrictive environments may underestimate the benefits of full autonomy. Faculty, preceptors, leaders, and individual APRNs share the responsibility to promote a vision of fully autonomous practice as a right and responsibility. It is critical that students, who are the profession's future, internalize a keen understanding of the importance of autonomy for both their practice and profession.

CONCLUSION

Imagine what APRN practice would be like if every state had fully autonomous practice and all APRNs embraced this autonomy. Changing laws is important, but changing the way we think about autonomy is even more important. "It is not just in action but in thought that we create our autonomy" (Kaplan & Brown, 2006, p. 37).

REFERENCES

Alabama Nurse Practice Act. (2006). Code of Alabama 1975, § 34-21-85. 610-X-5-.08 Amended 2006. Retrieved from http://www.abn.state.al.us/main/downloads/admin-code/chapter-610-X-5.html

American Medical Association. (2009). AMA scope of practice data series: Nurse practitioners. Retrieved from http://www.acnpweb.org/files/public/08-0424_SOP_Nurse_Revised_10_09.pdf

American Pain Society & American Academy of Pain Medicine. (2009). Guideline for the use of chronic opioid therapy in chronic noncancer pain: Evidence review. Retrieved from http://www.ampainsoc.org/pub/pdf/Opioid_Final_Evidence_Report.pdf

Americans United for Separation of Church and State. (2009). Retrieved from: http://www.au.org/what-we-do/lawsuits/archives/stormans-v-selecky.html

Brown, S. A., & Grimes, D. E. (1995). A meta-analysis of nurse practitioners and nurse midwives in primary care. *Nursing Research*, 44(6), 332–339.

Buppert, C. (2003). When is a medical doctor liable for nurse practitioner malpractice? *Medscape*.

Buppert, C. (2009). Can I order home health services for physician-ordered home healthcare? *Medscape*. Retrieved from http://www.medscape.com/viewarticle/703620

California Business and Professions Code. (2004). Chapter 6 Article 1 section 2836.1. Retrieved from http://www.rn.ca.gov/regulations/bpc.shtml#2836.1

Congressional Budget Office. (1979). *Physician extenders: Their current and future role in medical care delivery*. Washington, DC: US Government Printing Office.

Connecticut Department of Consumer Protection. (2009). Controlled Substance Registration. Title 21a Chapter 420c Sec. 21a-317. Retrieved from http://www.cga.ct.gov/2009/PUB/chap420c.htm

Drug Addiction Treatment Act of 2000. (2000). Public law 106-310-title XXXV Waiver authority for physicians who dispense or prescribe certain narcotic drugs for maintenance treatment or detoxification treatment. Retrieved from http://history.nih.gov/research/downloads/PL106-310.pdf

Dulisse, B., & Cromwell, J. (2010). No harm found when nurse anesthetists work without supervision by physicians.

Food and Drugs. (2005). Chapter II Drug Enforcement Administration, Department of Justice, Part 1306 Prescriptions. 21 CFR, Ch. II, §1306.07. Retrieved from http://edocket.access.gpo.gov/cfr_2010/aprqtr/pdf/21cfr1306.07.pdf

Georgia Board of Nursing. (2007) Laws, policies and rules. Retrieved from: http://sos.georgia.gov/plb/rn/

Georgia Board of Nursing Board Rules. (2008). Regulation of protocol use by advanced practice registered nurses as authorized by O.C.G.A §43-34-26.3 Chapter 410-13-.02 2(e) 1-6. Retrieved from http://rules.sos.state.ga.us/docs/410/13/02.pdf

Georgia Composite Medical Board. (2009). Medical Practice Act. §43-34-25 (d)-(e). Retrieved from http://medicalboard.georgia.gov/vgn/images/portal/cit_11783501/147915830Medical%20Practice%20Act%202009.pdf

Georgia Registered Professional Nurse Act. (2007). Definitions. §43-26-3. Retrieved from: http://sos.georgia.gov/plb/rn/

Hawkins, D. (2002). *Power vs. force: The hidden determinants of human behavior*. Australia: Hay House Publishing.

Horrocks, S., Anderson, E., & Salisbury, C. (2002). Systematic review of whether nurse practitioners working in primary care can provide equivalent care to doctors. *British Medical Journal, 324*(7341), 819–823.

Illinois Nursing and Advanced Practice Nursing Act. (2006). Title 68 Professions and occupations Chapter VII: Department of financial and professional regulation subchapter b: professions and occupations part 1305 nursing and advanced practice nursing act—advanced practice nurse section 1305.40 prescriptive authority. Retrieved from http://www.ilga.gov/commission/jcar/admincode/068/068013050000400R.html

Jenkins, S. M. (1994). The myth of vicarious liability. *Journal of Nurse Midwifery, 39*(2), 98–106.

Kaplan, L., & Brown, M. A. (2004). Prescriptive authority and barriers to NP practice. *Nurse Practitioner, 29*(3), 28–29, 32–35.

Kaplan, L., & Brown, M. A. (2006). What is "true" professional autonomy? *Nurse Practitioner, 31*(3), 37.

Kaplan, L., & Brown, M. A. (2008a). Prescribing controlled substances: Perceptions, realities, and experiences in Washington State. *American Journal for Nurse Practitioners*, 12(3), 41–51, 53.

Kaplan, L., & Brown, M. A. (2008b). Changing laws is not enough: Preparing ourselves for scope of practice changes. *American Journal for Nurse Practitioners*, 12(3), 52–53.

Kaplan, L., Brown, M. A., Andrilla, H., & Hart, L. G. (2006). Barriers to autonomous practice. *Nurse Practitioner*, 31(2), 57–63.

Kaplan, L., Brown, M. A., & Donahue, J. (2010). Prescribing controlled substances: How NPs in Washington are making a difference. *The Nurse Practitioner*, 35(5), 47–53.

Kaplan, L., Brown, M. A., & Simonson, D. (2011). CRNA prescribing practices: The Washington State experience. *AANA Journal*, 79(1), 24–29.

Kentucky Administrative Regulations 20:059. (2010). Section 1 Specific controlled substances. Retrieved from http://www.lrc. state.ky.us/kar/201/020/059.htm

Kentucky Revised Statutes. (2010). Chapter 314.011(8) Definitions for chapter "advanced practice registered nursing." Retrieved from http://162.114.4.13/KRS/314-00/011.PDF

Laurant, M., Reeves, D., Hermens, R., Braspenning, J., Grol, R., & Sibald, B. (2006). Substitution of doctors by nurses in primary care. *Cochrane Database Systematic Reviews*, (1).

Lenz, E. R., Mundinger, M. O., Kane, R. L., & Hopkins, S. C. (2002). Nurse practitioners and physician assistants in hospital outpatient departments, 1997–1999. *Nursing Economics*, 20(4), 174–179.

Lenz, E. R., Mundinger, M. O., Hopkins, S. C., & Lin, S. X. (2004). Primary care outcomes in patients treated by nurse practitioners or physicians: Two year follow-up. *Medical Care Research and Review*, 61(3), 332-351.

Michigan Nurses Association. (2009). Advanced practice nursing: Nurse practitioner frequently asked questions. Retrieved from http://www.minurses.org/APRN/APRN-npfaq.shtml

National Council of State Boards of Nursing. (2010). Member boards profiles. Retrieved from https://www.ncsbn.org/2010_Regulation_of_Advanced_Practice_Nursing.pdf

New Mexico Department of Health. (2009). Medical cannabis program. Retrieved from http://www.health.state.nm.us/idb/medical_cannabis.shtml

Newhouse, R. P., Stanik-Hutt, J., White, K. M., Johantgen, M., Bass, E., Zangaro, G., . . . Weiner, J. P. (2011). Advance practice nurse outcomes 1990–2008: A systematic review. *Nursing Economic$*, *29*(5), 1–22.

O'Grady, E. T., & Johnson, J. E. (2009). Health policy issues in changing environments. In A. B. Hamric, J. A. Spross, & C. M. Hanson (Eds.), *Advanced practice nursing: An integrative approach* (4th ed.). St. Louis, MO: Saunders Elsevier.

Ohio Administrative Code. (2009). Chapter 4731 state medical board 11-03 schedule II controlled substance stimulants and 11-04 controlled substances: Utilization for weight reduction. Retrieved from http://codes.ohio.gov/oac/4731-11

Ohio Board of Nursing. (2009). The formulary developed by the committee on prescriptive governance. Retrieved from http://www.nursing.ohio.gov/PDFS/AdvPractice/Formulary092109.pdf

Ohman-Strickland, P. A., Orzano, A. J., Hudson, S. V., Solberg, L. I., DiCiccio-Bloom, B., O'Malley, D., . . . Crabtree, B. F. (2008). Quality of diabetes care in family medicine practices: Influence of nurse-practitioners and physicians. *Annals of Family Medicine*, *6*(1), 14–22.

Pearson, L. (2011). The Pearson report. Retrieved from http://www.pearsonreport.com

Prescott, P. A., & Driscoll, L. (1980). Evaluating nurse practitioner performance. *Nurse Practitioner*, *1*(1), 28–32.

Public Health. (2003). Certification of opioid treatment programs. Chapter 1 Public Health Service, Department of Health and Human Services 42 CFR §8.12 6h. Retrieved from http://frwebgate.access.gpo.gov/cgi-bin/get-cfr.cgi

Safriet, B. J. (1992). Health care dollars and regulatory sense: The role of advanced practice nursing. *Yale Journal on Regulation*, *9*(2), 417–488.

Sherman, J. J., Fuller, S. G., & Hunter, S. G. (1999). Perceived barriers to prescriptive practices of advanced practice nurses. *Journal of the American Academy of Nurse Practitioners*, *11*(2), 63–68.

Simonson, D. C., Ahern, M. M., & Hendryx, M. S. (2007). Anesthesia staffing and anesthetic complications during cesarean delivery: A retrospective analysis. *Nursing Research*, *56*(1), 9–17.

Spitzer, W. O., Sackett, D. L., Sibley, J. C., Roberts, M., Gent, M., Kergin, D. J., . . . Olynich, A. (1974). The Burlington randomized trial of the nurse practitioner. *New England Journal of Medicine*, *290*(3), 252–256.

Take Care Clinics. (2010). Retrieved from http://takecarehealth. com/

Utah Nurse Practice Act. (2009). Title 58, chapter 31b-102 (13)(c) (iii). Retrieved from http://www.dopl.utah.gov/laws/58-31b. pdf

Wisconsin Administrative Code. (2000). Chapter N8 Certification of Advanced Practice Nurse Prescribers. N8.06(3)(a-f), N8.06(4). Retrieved from http://nxt.legis.state.wi.us/nxt/gateway.dll?f= templates&fn=default.htm&d=code&jd=ch.%20n%208

Strategies for Assessing, Monitoring, and Addressing Special Considerations with Controlled Substances

4

Pamela Stitzlein Davies

This chapter discusses deliberate, concrete approaches to building expertise in prescribing controlled substances (CSs). Approaches range from "universal precautions" for use with the prescription of CSs and the assessment and management of patients with chronic noncancer pain, to clinical guidelines, consensus statements, and practice standards for the identification of a patient who is at risk for substance abuse. Accurate definitions of terms related to drug use or misuse and their application create more skillful communication with patients around complex and sensitive issues.

Controlled substances (CSs) are powerful agents. When prescribed carefully, CSs can have a significant positive impact on quality of life, pain, function, mood, and sleep. When prescribed inappropriately, CSs use can be physically, emotionally, and socially harmful. It is important for the advanced practice registered nurse (APRN) to be a knowledgeable, competent, and astute prescriber of these drugs. Some APRNs choose not to prescribe CSs out of fear of

The Advanced Practice Registered Nurse as a Prescriber, First Edition. Marie Annette Brown, Louise Kaplan.
© 2012 John Wiley & Sons, Ltd. Published 2012 by John Wiley & Sons, Ltd.

adverse consequences and challenging situations. The analogy to fire is useful; fire can warm a house or burn it down.

When prescribing a CS, the APRN needs to consider several additional issues beyond the usual concerns related to prescribing. This chapter addresses special considerations related to patient assessment and monitoring, and reviews guidelines that facilitate the development of CS prescribing competencies.

CSS AND RELATED DEFINITIONS
Legend and controlled substances

Legend drugs refer to drugs that require a prescription. CSs are legend drugs regulated by the federal Controlled Substances Act of 1970 and have been determined to be a higher risk for abuse and diversion than other legend drugs. Prior to prescribing a CS, the health professional is required to register with the Drug Enforcement Administration (DEA). Schedule I drugs (e.g., heroin, marijuana) are illegal under federal law. Medical marijuana will not be addressed in this chapter. Schedule II drugs (e.g., morphine, fentanyl, methylphenidate) have been determined to have the highest abuse potential. The lower risk schedules are Schedule III (e.g., hydrocodone compounds/Vicodin®, testosterone), Schedule IV (e.g., butorphanol/Stadol®, diazepam, zolpidem), and Schedule V with the least potential for abuse (cough syrup with codeine, Lomotil®, pregabalin/Lyrica®).

Generally, these schedules reflect drug abuse potential. Occasionally, the assignment of a drug to a controlled status or schedule may seem somewhat unclear or confusing. For example, plain codeine is a Schedule II drug; in compounded form (Tylenol® #3), codeine is a Schedule III drug, while in Canada, low-dose codeine (8 mg) in combination with caffeine and acetaminophen or aspirin is available over-the-counter.

On the other hand, some legend drugs that are not federally classified as CS, such as carisoprodol (Soma®), have recently received closer scrutiny. Some states now regulate it as a Schedule III or IV drug due to the risk for abuse (Bramness & Skurtveit, 2008; Reeves & Burke, 2010). Norway has removed carisoprodol from the market entirely, and the European Medicines Agency has recommended it be withdrawn from all European Union member states due to abuse issues (Bramness, Furu, & Engeland, 2007).

Although tramadol (Ultram®) is not a CS, it may be sought by drug users and people with addiction disorders and is subject to criminal diversion (Food and Drug Administration, 2010). The abuse potential may warrant reclassifying it as a CS in the future (Drug Enforcement Administration [DEA], 2009). Interestingly, tapentadol (Nucynta®), which is similar in structure to tramadol, was FDA-approved in 2009 as a Schedule II drug.

Definitions

It is critical to correctly define terms related to drug use or misuse. Box 4.1 lists commonly used definitions. These definitions were endorsed in a 2001 consensus statement developed by the American

---

Box 4.1 Definitions related to controlled drug use

Abuse: "Any use of an illegal drug, or the intentional self-administration of a medication for nonmedical purpose such as altering one's state of consciousness, for example, getting high" (Chou et al., 2009, p. 130).

Aberrant drug-related behavior: "A behavior outside the boundaries of the agreed on treatment plan which is established as early as possible" (Chou et al., 2009, p. 130).

Addiction: "Addiction is a primary, chronic disease of brain reward, motivation, memory and related circuitry. Dysfunction in these circuits leads to characteristic biological, psychological, social and spiritual manifestations. This is reflected in an individual pathologically pursuing reward and/or relief by substance use and other behaviors.

"Addiction is characterized by inability to consistently abstain, impairment in behavioral control, craving, diminished recognition of significant problems with one's behaviors and interpersonal relationships, and a dysfunctional emotional response. Like other chronic diseases, addiction often involves cycles of relapse and remission. Without treatment or engagement in recovery activities, addiction is progressive and can result in disability or premature death" (American Society of Addiction Medicine, 2001).

Chemical coping: "describes a patient who uses pain medicines to alleviate non-pain symptoms, such as anxiety or depression" (Nabati & Abrahm, 2008, p. 322).

Diversion: "The intentional transfer of a controlled substance from legitimate distribution and dispensing channels" (Chou et al., 2009, p. 130).

Continued

Habituation: "a less intense attachment that occur(s) in response to drugs which never produce compulsive craving, yet their pharmacologic action is found desirable to some individuals who readily form a habit of administration" (Savage, 2008, p. 10).

Misuse: "use of a medication (for a medical purpose) other than as directed or as indicated, whether willful or unintentional, and whether harm results or not" (Chou et al., 2009 p. 130).

Narcotic: "a legal term referring to a number of illicit substances including heroin and cocaine. The use of the term *narcotic* should be discouraged when reference to opioid medications is intended" (Savage, 2008, p. 12).

Opiates: "Drugs that are derived from opium, either natural or semisynthetic opioids. The DEA and other agencies refer to all opioids, even synthetic drugs, as '*opiates*'" (Savage, 2008, p. 12).

Opioid: "Meaning 'opium-like' an inclusive term referring to all drugs that act as opioid receptors in the central and peripheral nervous systems. These include naturally occurring drugs (morphine, heroin), semi-synthetic drugs (oxycodone, hydrocodone), and synthetic drugs (fentanyl, methadone). This is a more accurate term than opiate or narcotic" (Savage, 2008, pp. 11–12).

Physical dependence: "a state of adaptation that is manifested by a drug class specific withdrawal syndrome that can be produced by abrupt cessation, rapid dose reduction, decreasing blood level of the drug, and/or administration of an antagonist" (American Academy of Pain Medicine, American Pain Society, & American Society of Addiction Medicine, 2001).

Pseudoaddiction: "The iatrogenic syndrome of abnormal behavior developing as a direct consequence of inadequate pain management" (Weissman & Haddox, 1989).

Substance use: "a maladaptive pattern of drug use behavior leading to significant impairment or distress, such as failure to fulfill major role obligations at home, work or in school. To meet DSM-IV criteria, this must be demonstrated for at least 12 months" (Savage, 2008, p. 10).

Tolerance: "a state of adaptation in which exposure to a drug induces changes that result in a diminution of one or more of the drug's effects over time" (American Academy of Pain Medicine, American Pain Society, & American Society of Addiction Medicine, 2001).

Academy of Pain Medicine, the American Pain Society, and the American Society of Addiction Medicine. Improper use of terms creates confusion. For example, clinicians commonly but incorrectly use the term "addiction" instead of "tolerance" to describe normal and expected adaptation to chronic use of a CS. The correct definition of addiction is "behaviors that include one or more of the following: impaired control over drug use, compulsive use, continued use despite harm, and craving." The terms tolerance, physical dependence, and addiction (more appropriately called psychological dependence) are of central importance. It is essential for APRNs to use terms appropriately to assure that professional communication and documentation is accurate. This also assures that patients are educated about the benefits and risks of CSs. A particularly good "teachable moment" can occur when patients comment "I don't want to become addicted." Helping them understand the differences between addiction and physiological or psychological dependence can be reassuring. Additionally, APRNs should routinely use the term "opioid" instead of "narcotic," as the former refers to synthetic as well as naturally occurring drugs that have effects similar to opium and opium derivatives (Savage, 2008; Stedman, 2006).

THE "DECADE OF PAIN CONTROL" VERSUS THE "WAR ON DRUGS"
Decade of Pain

Out of concern to improve the lives of people who live with pain, Congress passed a law in 2000 which declared a "Decade of Pain Control and Research." The goals were to raise awareness, improve treatment, and increase funding for research on pain. This decade saw many advances in the neuroscience of pain, new technologies for diagnosis and treatment of pain, and emergence of the role of complementary medicine in pain management (Boswell & Giordano, 2009). Concurrently, The Joint Commission (2010) issued standards in 2001 recognizing that every patient has the right to appropriate assessment and management of pain. Pain management moved to the forefront and pain became known as "the 5th vital sign."

The Decade of Pain Control and Research directly lead to inclusion of some of the provisions from the National Pain Care Policy Act of 2009 into healthcare reform legislation in 2010. The legislation mandated an Institute of Medicine conference on pain; charged the National Institutes of Health with development of a Pain Consortium for ongoing pain research; and directed the Department of Health and Human Services to develop a program to enhance health professionals' expertise in pain management and increase the utilization of comprehensive pain care centers (American Academy of Pain Medicine, 2010).

The Decade of Pain Control and Research also endeavored to replace the fear, avoidance, and stigmatization of "narcotics" with acceptance and even encouragement to prescribe opioids for cancer and chronic noncancer pain. This was in stark contrast to other approaches that began as early as 1954 when the Eisenhower administration created a Cabinet committee "to stamp out narcotic addiction." The Nixon administration continued this momentum in the 1969 "War on Drugs," the passage of the Comprehensive Drug Abuse Prevention and Control Act of 1970, and the creation of the DEA in 1973 (Suddath, 2009).

Scott Fishman (2007), past president of the American Academy of Pain Medicine, states "the collision between the *War on Pain* and the *War on Drugs* has created a 'perfect storm' of controversy" (p. 5). Unfortunately, prescription drug abuse has risen to a crisis point, yet many believe that pain is still undertreated (Boswell & Giordano, 2009).

Prescription drug abuse

Abuse of prescription drugs, especially opioids, is a growing problem in the United States. The Drug Abuse Warning Network (DAWN), which monitors drug-related deaths and drug-related visits to emergency departments (EDs), reported an estimated 4.3 million visits from 2004 to 2008 (a 97% increase) for the nonmedical use of pharmaceuticals. ED visits involving central nervous system agents represented 74% of the visits with 47% related to pain relievers (Drug Abuse Warning Network [DAWN], 2011, p. 10). The medications most responsible for these visits were oxycodone (105,214 visits), hydrocodone (89,051 visits), methadone (63,629 visits), and other opiates/opioids (66,585 visits) (DAWN, 2011, p. 46.). Also of note were 325,041 benzodiazepine-related visits (DAWN, 2011). There has been a steady increase in abuse of oral prescription opioids, especially among teens and young adults (Comer & Ashworth, 2008; National Drug Intelligence Center,

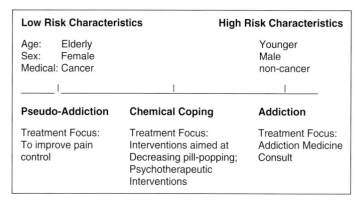

Fig. 4.1 Spectrum of problematic drug use behaviors and risk characteristics. *Source*: Reprinted from Passik & Kirsh 2008, Chemical coping: The clinical middle ground. In Howard S. Smith and Steven D Passik (Eds.) *Pain and Chemical Dependency*, with permission from Oxford University Press, Inc.

2009). The most popular supply of drugs to abuse is found in the home medicine cabinet (Webster & Dove, 2007). Deaths related to prescription drug abuse have surpassed motor vehicle deaths in some states such as Washington (Agency Medical Directors Group [AMDG], 2010).

The risk of drug abuse should be thought as a spectrum. Lower risk individuals are more likely to be older in age, female, and receiving medications for cancer-related pain (Fig. 4.1). In addition, they typically have a minimal substance use history and are non-smokers. Higher risk individuals are younger, male, and have a noncancer diagnosis. Additionally, they are likely to be smokers with a significant past or current history of substance use and psychopathology. Passik and Kirsh (2008) describe a *chemical coper* who fits in the middle of the abuse spectrum. These are persons who occasionally use their medications in a nonprescribed manner as a way of coping with stress. They are focused on obtaining drugs, and are inflexible and uninterested in pursuing other treatment options for pain.

RECOMMENDED PRACTICES FOR PRESCRIBERS OF CONTROLLED SUBSTANCES

Universal precautions in pain medicine

It is impossible to determine with accuracy which clients will develop problems with CSs. Gourlay, Heit, and Almahrezi (2005) proposed the concept of "Universal Precautions in Pain Medicine" (Box 4.2). This is similar to preventing the transmission of infectious disease by *always* wearing gloves when at risk of contact with bodily fluids.

Initially designed for opioid prescribing, the concept can be utilized when prescribing all CSs. Universal precautions are a standard-

---

Box 4.2 Universal precautions in pain medicine

1. Make a diagnosis, identify treatable causes of pain
2. Perform a psychological assessment including risk of addictive disorders
3. Discuss urine drug testing with all patients
4. Informed consent: benefits and risks of treatment
5. Verbal or written treatment agreement reviewing the expectations and obligations of both the prescriber and the patient
6. Emphasize that opioid therapy is initially a *therapeutic trial* based on clinical goals
7. Have a rational plan for appropriate use of opioid therapy and adjunctive medications
8. Regular reassessment of pain score and level of function Corroborate with third parties if possible
9. Regularly assess the "5 A's" of pain medicine
    a. Analgesia
    b. Activity
    c. Adverse effects
    d. Aberrant behavior
    e. Affect
10. Periodically review the patient's diagnosis and comorbid conditions, including addictive disorders
11. Documentation of initial and ongoing assessments

Source: Gourlay et al., 2005.

---

ized approach toward *all patients* receiving long-term opioid prescriptions and other CSs. They create an unbiased method of protecting both the patient and the prescriber of CSs. Key points include assessing the risk of addictive disorders in all patients, forming a treatment agreement with an emphasis on an initial therapeutic trial of the drug, regular reassessment, and documentation.

A helpful clinical tool related to universal precautions is the "5 A's of Pain Medicine" with the elements analgesia, activity, adverse effects, aberrant behavior, and affect (Gourlay et al., 2005). Use of the 5 A's includes inquiring about aspects of each element: analgesia—pain intensity, pain relief; activity—reaching functional goals; adverse effects—constipation, sedation, cognitive changes, pruritus; aberrant behavior—inappropriate use of a CS or sharing drugs; and affect—mood, perceived personality changes. These five areas are essential for proper assessment when prescribing an opioid. Additionally, the 5 A's provide easy cues for comprehensive, yet brief, documentation.

Assessment of patient status with the 5 A's has been discussed in the opioid therapy literature but not in respect to other CSs. Clinicians may also find it useful to assess the impact of benzodiazepines, stimulants, hypnotics, and other CSs with this brief tool by substituting "analgesia" with "anxiety," "agitation," "hyperactivity," or "sleep."

As part of universal precautions, it is recommended that the primary care provider stratify patients in the initial assessment into three levels of care. The levels are based on the risk for aberrant behavior related to use of CSs including opioids, benzodiazepines, and stimulants. Placing a patient in a particular level reflects the APRN's expectation of who will provide the care and what kind of collaboration would likely be the most appropriate. Each level increases the need for collaborative care or specialty referral according to patient characteristics. These levels are:

Level 1: Primary Care
Level 2: Primary Care with Specialist Support
Level 3: Specialty Pain Management

This stratification process is not meant to be punitive or perpetuate stereotypes. The goals are to keep the patient and prescriber safe, diagnose treatable conditions such as depression, and maintain clinical practice within standards of care.

Level 1, *Primary Care*, represents the lowest risk patient with no personal or family history of alcohol or drug abuse, and no major or untreated psychopathology. The majority of patients who present to the primary care APRN are in this category. Level 2, *Primary Care with Specialist Support*, includes patients with a past personal or family history of substance use; current psychopathology including untreated or poorly controlled depression or anxiety; or major psychopathology such as schizophrenia or personality disorder. These patients are at moderate risk of inappropriate drug-related behaviors. The primary care APRN is encouraged to consult formally or informally with a specialist when providing CSs prescriptions to Level 2 patients. Level 3, *Specialty Pain Management*, encompasses people with active substance abuse or severe untreated psychopathology who are at high risk of aberrant behaviors related to use of CSs. Most primary care providers lack the experience, resources, and skills to care for these complex patients and should refer their care to a multidisciplinary comprehensive pain management specialist (Chou et al., 2009; Gourlay et al., 2005).

Referral is hindered in many communities and patient populations by an insufficient number of specialists. Often, weeks or months are required to obtain an appointment for a patient evaluation. This creates a special challenge for the primary care APRN in need of assistance with a complex patient. APRNs are encouraged to identify colleagues with expertise in pain management, addiction, psychiatry, and sleep medicine with whom they can consult. Additionally, APRNs with expertise in pain management are encouraged to be available as resources to their colleagues.

Certification in pain management specific to nurse practitioners or advance practice nurses is not currently available. The American Society for Pain Management Nursing (ASPMN, aspmn.org) offers Pain Management Nursing Certification to registered nurses. However, as of fall 2011, there are no plans to create a certification exam which is specific to advance practice nurses. The American Academy of Pain Management (AAPM, aapainmanage.org) offers a "Credentialed Pain Practitioner" to any healthcare provider who has worked in the pain field for 2 years. The exam is the same for all healthcare disciplines. As of fall 2011, the cost for AAPM credentialing was $1075. The Hospice and Palliative Nurses Association (hpna.org) in conjunction with the National Board for Certification of Hospice and Palliative Nurses (NBCHPN(R)) offers certification as an Advanced Certified Hospice and Pallia- tive Nurse (ACHPN®), which includes topics on pain manage- ment in the exam. ASPMN, in partnership with the American Nurses Credentialing Center, offers *Pain Management Nursing Certification.*

In summary, use of universal precautions for CSs with *all* patients, triaging to the appropriate risk category, implementing a plan based on risk category and reassessing patients regularly, reduces the risk of prescribing CSs to an unidentified active abuser. Consistent use of universal precautions assists in the early detec- tion of aberrant behaviors. Patients may express concern that they are being stigmatized and should be reassured that *all* individuals who are prescribed CSs on a long-term basis are screened in a similar manner. The discussions will likely be most effective when approached with mutual trust and respect (Gourlay and Heit 2006) (see Box 4.3)

Box 4.3 Case example: stratifying a patient for opioid misuse under universal precautions in pain medicine

Susan Butler, APRN, meets with Ms. Jones who presents for a new patient visit accompanied by her adult son who is also your patient. Ms. Jones is a 68-year-old woman who just moved to the area to live with her son's family. She is a widow who lived alone but is becoming frail and has fallen twice. She is neatly groomed, very pleasant, with good eye contact, but with mild cognitive deficit apparent upon detailed history taking. Ms. Jones reports pain from moderately severe osteoar- thritis in her hips, knees, and fingers. She brings records from her out- of-state primary care provider showing she has been maintained on oxycodone CR 20 mg BID and oxycodone 5 mg for breakthrough pain for several years. There are no problematic drug-taking behaviors noted in the brief progress notes.

Continued

Despite many cues that Ms. Jones represents a low-risk patient for opioid prescriptions, and with concerns that it may offend this dignified older woman, the APRN nonetheless asks the standard screening questions about substance use and psychosocial history. She is surprised to discover that Ms. Jones drinks excessive quantities of alcohol based on her gender and age, reporting four to five shots of rum on weekends, and two to three shots on weekday nights. This is reduced from two-fifths of rum nightly for decades. With a twinkle in her eye, she states: "I was a bartender. The rules are different when you work in a bar. You *have* to drink!" She also has a 100 pack year smoking history, reduced to one-half pack per day in the last 2 years. Ms. Jones reports her estranged adult daughter has an active substance use disorder for over a decade: "She takes any drug she can get her hands on." Ms. Jones also has depression and poorly treated anxiety since her husband died several years ago. She admits to occasionally taking opioids for anxiety management and sleep problems which caused her to use the allotted number pills before refills were due and request additional medication.

Based on the universal precautions stratification system reported above, the APRN stratifies the patient to Level 3, *Specialty Pain Management*, due to active alcohol abuse. She has a frank discussion with the patient and her son, telling them that in her professional opinion, the risks of opioids outweigh the benefits. She therefore declines to prescribe ongoing opioid therapy. The APRN emphasizes her commitment to help manage Ms. Jones' pain and describes other treatment options available based on the American Geriatrics Society guidelines on persistent pain. She expresses concern about patient safety and fall risk, given the concurrent use of alcohol and opioids. She gently addresses the patient's dismissal of concerns about alcohol intake. Ms. Jones agrees to see a pain specialist but declines a separate referral to an addiction specialist. However, with her son's input, she reluctantly agrees that she is probably drinking too much "for my age," and agrees to "cut down" on her intake. She does not agree to stop drinking or to attend Alcoholics Anonymous meetings because she does not believe she has a significant problem. She agrees to a trial of an antidepressant to aid in anxiety management and sleep.

Ms. Jones reports she only has 5 days of opioids left, and shows her the nearly empty prescription bottles.

What would you do at this point? There is more than one correct answer. Several possibilities include the following.

1. Maintain her current prescription of oxycodone CR, but stop the short-acting oxycodone, and follow-up every 2 weeks for several visits to assess her status and develop a new plan.

2. Refer the patient to her previous provider, who might be willing to prescribe the opioids until the first available pain clinic visit.
3. Taper and discontinue the CS.

In this case, Ms. Butler, the APRN, concerned about safety with this patient on opioids, decided to taper Ms. Jones off opioids over 10–14 days. A small supply of reduced-dose opioids was given to prevent withdrawal symptoms, and detailed written instructions were provided. Ms. Butler also prescribed other analgesics. Because it is likely that an appointment with the pain management clinic may not be available for 6 weeks, she arranges for Ms. Jones to return in 10 days.

Clinical guidelines and consensus statements

Familiarity with major professional association guidelines and consensus statements related to CSs will keep the APRN informed of current practice standards. For example, the American Pain Society and American Academy of Pain Medicine published *Clinical Guidelines for the Use of Chronic Opioid Therapy in Chronic Noncancer Pain* in 2009 (Box 4.4) (Chou et al., 2009). By following these 14 recommendations, the APRN can prescribe opioids for chronic noncancer pain in a judicious manner while recognizing patient behaviors that warrant closer monitoring, consultation, or discontinuation of the medications.

The guidelines contain tools for assessment of pain and risk of opioid misuse. Several screening tools, which are mentioned in this and other guidelines, include the Pain Assessment and Documentation Tool (PADT), the Opioid Risk Tool (ORT), the Screener and Opioid Assessment for Persons with Pain (SOAPP), the Diagnosis, Intractability, Risk Efficacy (DIRE) scale, the Current Opioid Misuse Measure (COMM), as well as a sample opioid agreement.

The Canadian Pain Society updated practice guidelines on chronic opioid therapy (COT) for noncancer pain (Furlan, Reardon, Weppler, & National Opioid Use Guideline Group, 2010). The 24 recommendations are grouped into three major categories: deciding to initiate opioid therapy; conducting a trial of opioid therapy; and monitoring long-term opioid therapy. Unique to this guideline is a protocol for tapering benzodiazepines prior to initiating COT

Box 4.4 Clinical guidelines for the use of chronic opioid therapy in chronic noncancer pain

(from the American Pain Society and American Academy of Pain Medicine)

1. **Patient selection and risk stratification:**
   The clinician should conduct a history and physical examination, perform appropriate diagnostic testing, and determine risk stratification for aberrant behaviors.

2. **Informed consent and opioid management plans:**
   Informed consent should be obtained. Consider using a written management plan for informed consent. Counsel patients that "total pain relief is rare," pain improvement is usually in the range of 20%–30%. Discuss goals of therapy and indications to continue or stop therapy.

3. **Initiation and titration of chronic opioid therapy:**
   Counsel the patient to consider the initial treatment period as a therapeutic trial. Drug selection, dosing, and titration should be individualized.

4. **Methadone:**
   Clinicians should become familiar with the complicated and variable pharmacokinetics and pharmacodynamics of methadone prior to prescribing.

5. **Monitoring:**
   Reassess patients periodically and document pain intensity, level of functioning, progress toward goals, adverse effects, and adherence to therapy. Consider performing urine drug screens.

6. **High-risk patients:**
   Patients at high risk for aberrant drug-related behavior require more frequent and vigilant monitoring. Consult mental health or addiction specialist for higher risk patients.

7. **Dose escalations, high-dose opioid therapy, opioid rotation, and indications for discontinuation of therapy:**
   Repeated dose escalations warrant reassessment of benefit to harm ratio. Doses over 200 mg daily of oral morphine (or equivalent) should trigger more frequent and intense monitoring, and consider opioid rotation. Patients should be tapered off opioids if they are engaging in serious or ongoing aberrant drug-related behaviors.

8. **Opioid-related adverse effects:**
   Clinicians should anticipate, counsel patients, identify, and treat common opioid side effects including constipation.

9. **Use of psychotherapeutic co-interventions:**
   Integrate psychotherapeutic and counseling interventions, functional restoration, interdisciplinary therapy, and other adjunctive nonopioid therapies (e.g., acupuncture) into the care plan.
10. **Driving and work safety:**
    Clinicians should counsel patients about cognitive effects on driving and work safety and provide appropriate guidelines or restrictions.
11. **Identifying a healthcare home and when to obtain consultation:**
    Patients should identify a clinician who coordinates care for the patient. Clinicians should seek consultation when additional skills or resources are needed to address the patient's needs.
12. **Breakthrough pain:**
    Consider adding short-acting, as-needed medications for brief episodes of worsening pain.
13. **Opioids in pregnancy:**
    Counsel women of childbearing age of the risks and benefits of opioids during pregnancy, and minimize use.
14. **Opioid policies:**
    Clinicians should be aware of current federal and state laws, regulatory guidelines, and policy statements that govern medical use of chronic opioid therapy for chronic noncancer pain.

Source: Chou et al., 2009.

to decrease the risk of sedation and overdose, especially in the elderly.

The American Geriatrics Society Panel on Pharmacological Management of Persistent Pain in Older Persons (2009) provided updated guidelines in August 2009. This guideline focuses on age-associated changes in drug metabolism which place older adults at higher risk for adverse drug reactions. Particular attention is given to nonsteroidal anti-inflammatory drugs (NSAIDs) and opioids in the elderly. Risk stratification for aberrant behaviors is reviewed, with reference to universal precautions and screening tools.

The Veterans Administration (VA) and Department of Defense (DoD) have been pioneers in the pain field, with the VA being the first large organization to institute use of *Pain as the 5th Vital Sign* (Geriatrics and Extended Care Strategic Healthcare Group, 2000). An updated Clinical Practice Guideline, "Management of Opioid Therapy for Chronic Pain," was issued by the VA/DoD in May 2010 (The Management of Opioid Therapy for Chronic Pain Working Group, 2010). The guideline contains a wealth of information the primary care provider will find useful in daily practice. Their unique strength is the detailed information about the management of complex populations and those at higher risk of aberrant drug behavior. The algorithms may assist the APRN who treats similar high-risk populations. This resource provides excellent guidance for the APRN's choice of opioid therapy in special populations such as people with renal and hepatic dysfunction, seizure risk, elderly, and decreased CYP-2D6 metabolism.

The Federation of State Medical Boards (2010) website has compiled *Resources for Pharmacovigilance and Pain Management*. Important on this site is the "Model Policy for the Use of Controlled Substances for the Treatment of Pain" (Federation of State Medical Boards (2004) (Box 4.5). The resources include links to other sites, several of which are sponsored by pharmaceutical companies and contain clinician and patient education materials and screening tools.

Several states have developed guidelines for use of COT for patients with chronic noncancer pain. The Washington State Agency Medical Directors Group (AMDG) released an updated guideline in May 2010. The website also offers the *Opioid Dosing Calculator* for calculation of daily morphine equivalent doses. The Utah Department of Health has an extensive guideline on opioid therapy. This 2009 guideline includes information on opioid management of acute pain as well as chronic pain.

Guidelines for the use of other CSs, such as benzodiazepines or stimulants, are not available at this time. However, Schutte-Rodin, Broch, Buysse, Dorsey, and Sateia (2008) have developed the "Clinical Guideline for the Evaluation and Management of Chronic Insomnia in Adults." This gives the primary care provider a general approach to prescribing insomnia medications, including suggested sequences of selecting drugs. However, the guideline does not address management of inappropriate or problematic behaviors related to hypnotic use.

Box 4.5 Model policy for the use of controlled substances for the treatment of pain

The *Model Policy for Use of Controlled Substances for the Treatment of Pain* was adopted in 1998 and updated in 2004 by the Federation of State Medical Boards with the goal of promoting consistency in state medical board policy. As of March 2008, 32 states have adopted the Policy in whole or in part (Pain & Policy Studies Group, 2008, p. 15).
  Guidelines

1. Evaluation of the patient
   Health history and physical exam must be obtained and documented in the medical record, along with the medical indication for treatment with a controlled substance (CS).
2. Treatment plan
   A written treatment plan should state objectives that will determine treatment success, such as pain relief, improved physical and psychosocial function.
3. Informed consent and agreement for treatment
   Discuss risks and benefits of use of CSs. Prescriptions should be from one provider and one pharmacy when possible. Consider use of a written agreement.
4. Periodic Review
   Periodically review the course of pain treatment for progress or lack of progress toward treatment goals.
5. Consultation
   Refer the patient for additional evaluation and treatment in order to reach treatment objectives. Special attention should be given to those patients at risk for medication misuse, abuse, or diversion.
6. Health Records
   Keep accurate records to include the above-listed items. In addition, records should include medications prescribed, instructions, treatment agreements.
7. Compliance with Controlled Substances Laws and Regulations
   The provider must be licensed and comply with applicable federal and state regulations.

The APRN is advised to stay current with federal and state rules related to prescribing of CSs. Guidelines from professional, federal, or state organizations can provide direction and a framework for approaching the patient who may require a CS prescription.

APPROACHES TO ASSESSMENT AND MANAGEMENT

The importance of a thorough patient assessment as the basis for creating a diagnosis and plan of care cannot be overemphasized. Long-term prescribing of CSs entails the review of factors beyond the patient's initial symptom that prompted the treatment. The assessment of the risk of misuse or diversion of the prescribed CS is also included.

Assessment of the patient

A comprehensive pain history will include not only assessment of the primary symptom (pain location, intensity, character, exacerbating and relieving factors, radiation, temporal factors), but will also address the impact of pain on mood, sleep, work, relationships, sexuality, recreation, and general functioning. A similar approach can be useful for patients using CSs for other problems such as anxiety disorders, insomnia, and hyperactivity. This information can be obtained through interview as well as self-administered questionnaires. The Washington State AMDG opioid guidelines contain several tools that can be used to assess patients including the ORT and the CAGE-AID (CAGE Adapted to Include Drugs). The Brief Pain Inventory can be used to assess the severity of a patient's pain and the impact of pain on the patient's life (Cleeland & Ryan, 1994).

When obtaining a patient history, inquire about personal or family history of smoking, alcohol, substance use, and psychiatric problems such as significant depression, anxiety, schizophrenia, and personality disorder. Affirmative responses stratify the patient to a higher risk category for CS misuse. It is also important to obtain and review records from previous providers because past behavior is predictive of future behavior in respect to CS use or misuse (Chou, 2010).

Physical examination should address the specific complaint, such as a neurological exam for complaints of headache, or spine palpation, range of motion, and gait for low back pain. The provider should also consider examination of additional systems to detect comorbid conditions that may contribute to the need for CSs or impact prescribing (e.g., presence of sleep apnea will impact the dose of opioid or benzodiazepine prescribed).

Assess for signs of drug abuse, such as:

- Track marks—scars from needle use in the antecubital space or other sites of venous access in the arms, legs, or neck
- Skin popping—scars from subcutaneous injection of drugs
- Nasal septal perforation from cocaine use
- Mentation changes such as nodding off during the visit from medication over sedation and unexpectedly small or large pupil size.

The diagnosis should be as specific as possible based on findings in the history, physical examination, and diagnostic tests. For example, spinal stenosis or myofascial tenderness is preferred over the generic term "back pain."

Lab testing

Use of routine urine drug testing (UDT) in primary care remains controversial but is gaining wider acceptance, and can be helpful in decision making prior to initiating a CS prescription and for ongoing surveillance. The purpose of UDT is to supplement patient self-report by identifying drug use related to illicit drugs or drugs not prescribed for the patient to verify the agreed-upon treatment program is followed. Most of the guidelines previously cited recommend consideration of UDT, especially if the patient has a history of higher risk behaviors. Surprisingly, a study by Katz et al. (2003) showed that 21% of patients on COT, who demonstrated no behavioral issues, had unexpected positive drug screens for either an illicit drug or nonprescribed controlled medication. They concluded: "Our results suggest that all patients receiving long-term opioid treatment for noncancer pain should be monitored with urine toxicology testing" (p. 1101). For that reason, some clinics perform UDT on all patients receiving COT, as part of universal precautions.

There are two primary urine drug tests available, the "point-of-service" dipstick or rapid test and the comprehensive laboratory conducted test. The "point-of-service" test costs $10–$50 and typically includes the "NIDA 5" (National Institute of Drug Abuse): cannabinoids (marijuana), cocaine, amphetamines, opiates (naturally including only-heroin, opium, codeine, morphine), and phencyclidine (PCP). NIDA-5 tests do not detect synthetic or semisynthetic opioids (oxycodone, hydrocodone, fentanyl, meperidine), benzodiazepines, or barbiturates. However, test results are available within minutes. Positive results must be confirmed by a comprehensive test as some agents can cause false-positive results.

Comprehensive UDT assesses for most of the commonly used scheduled drugs including benzodiazepines and barbiturates. It tests for opioids (synthetic or semisynthetic such as hydromorphone, hydrocodone, meperidine) as well as opiates (naturally occurring, such as morphine). The initial screen is an immunoassay, with confirmatory testing performed with gas chromatography/ mass spectrometry (GC/MS). Depending on the lab, oxycodone, fentanyl, and methadone may or may not be included in a comprehensive test. Some labs require that testing for these drugs be specifically requested. The provider must become familiar with the requirements of the individual toxicology lab for specifics on testing requests. It takes several days to obtain results and costs $100–$300. The comprehensive UDT is not always covered by insurance. Opioids can be detected in the urine during up to 3–4 days after ingestion (AMDG, 2010; Carlozzi et al., 2008).

UDT can be confusing to interpret. An understanding of pharmacokinetics, drug metabolism, and limitations of testing is needed (Chou et al., 2009). Therefore, an ongoing consultative relationship with the laboratory toxicologist will aid in proper interpretation of test results. For example, codeine is metabolized to small quantities of morphine and hydrocodone. A patient prescribed codeine may appropriately have small amounts of these drugs found in the UDT. Likewise, oxycodone has minor metabolism to oxymorphone and that substance may be detected in the UDT (Carlozzi et al., 2008; Webster & Dove, 2007) (see Table 4.1).

The APRN needs to consider what drugs may be used by the patient when choosing between the "point of service" and comprehensive test. The "point-of-service" test will not reveal presence of synthetic opioids such as oxycodone or fentanyl. Patients are sometimes accused of not taking a prescribed drug, when, in fact, the drug cannot be detected by the particular test performed. Likewise, unsanctioned drug use may not be detected if the rapid test is performed. For example, a rapid "dipstick" UDT will not detect

Table 4.1 Interpreting urine drug screens: selected opioid metabolites

Drug	Urinary metabolites
Morphine	Morphine, hydromorphone, codeine
Codeine	Codeine, morphine, hydrocodone
Hydrocodone	Hydrocodone, hydromorphone
Oxycodone	Oxycodone, oxymorphone, hydrocodone

Source: Adapted from Webster and Dove (2007, p. 142).

illicit use of oxycodone (Webster & Dove, 2007). The APRN should consult with the laboratory toxicology technician to confirm interpretation of unexpected findings prior to discussing the results with a patient or making any changes in therapy based on test results. Washington State's AMDG guidelines have extensive information on UDT in the appendix, including information on interpretation of test results, decision algorithms, and UDT clinical vignettes.

Additional lab testing

As with any drug, the clinician should assess for renal or hepatic compromise prior to prescribing a CS. Consideration should be given to testing for hepatitis B, hepatitis C, and HIV for any patient with a history of illicit drug use.

CS agreements

Prior to prescribing CSs on a long-term basis, the expectations and responsibilities of the APRN and patient need to be clearly delineated, communicated, and documented. The APRN also needs to explain the consequences if patient expectations and responsibilities are unmet. Utilizing a written treatment agreement can facilitate this process. This is most commonly done with patients on COT with chronic noncancer pain. The documents may have titles such as Opioid Agreement, Opioid Care Plan, or Informed Consent for Chronic Opioid Therapy (previously referred to as "Narcotic Contract"). Examples are available in the appendices of the American Pain Society guidelines for use of COT in chronic noncancer pain and the Washington State AMDG guidelines. The agreements can be adapted for use with other CSs such as benzodiazepines or sedative hypnotics (Ciraulo & Ciraulo, 2008).

Typically included in the written opioid care plan agreement are expectations specifying that the patient will obtain CS prescriptions from only one provider or provider group and will fill them at only one pharmacy. Some providers may also include the requirement to abstain from drinking alcohol or smoking marijuana while taking the CS. The agreement can function as an educational tool about the management of possible drug side effects such as constipation or sedation, driving safety, drug safekeeping in the home, and avoiding drug interactions. It can be used to instruct patients on clinic policies such as two business days are needed for renewals, no renewals on evenings or weekends, no replacement of lost or stolen prescriptions, or random urine drug screens will be performed. This standardized approach provides consistency and should be applied to all patients. Box 4.6 describes items commonly included in CS agreements.

PRESCRIBING CONTROLLED SUBSTANCES
Initiating CS prescriptions

When starting a patient on a new CS prescription, consider providing only a 2-week supply with a follow-up in 2 weeks. If no concerning behaviors develop, quantities can be increased to a 30-day supply with or without refills, and visits extended to 1–3 months. Although there are no specific guidelines for frequency of visits, most providers see patients who are stable on chronic opioid or other CS therapy once every 1–3 months and at a minimum every 6 months (AMDG, 2010; Department of Veterans Affairs & Department of Defense, 2010).

According to federal law, it is legal to prescribe an unlimited amount of CSs. However, some states may impose quantity restrictions of CSs, as will some insurance companies. Most providers limit quantities of CSs to a 30-day supply because of concern about theft or risk of overdose. However, a 90-day supply of CSs may be more convenient and decrease the financial burden on patients. A 90-day supply may also be appropriate for people who require long-term CS therapy and who are stable and responsible. The APRN will need to determine the individual's risk for misuse or loss when considering a prescription for larger quantities of CSs.

Box 4.6 Items typically included in an opioid agreement

Informed consent

- Goals of opioid treatment
- Risks and benefits of opioid treatment
- Alternatives to opioid treatment

Expectations

- One prescriber of opioids, do not obtain opioids from other offices
- Allow three business days for renewal requests
- Use only one pharmacy
- Keep follow-up appointments
- See physical therapy and other referrals as requested
- Honesty regarding history of substance use
- Random urine drug screens and pill counts
- Progress toward functional goals

Patient education

- Use only as prescribed
- Expected side effects
- Management of side effects
- When and where to call for questions or problems
- Driving safety and work safety related to cognitive changes
- Do not share with others
- Keep drugs locked in a safe place to avoid them being stolen (even by family or acquaintances)
- Treat the prescription and opioid pills like cash, do not leave them out
- No refills on evenings or weekends
- "No early refill" policy
- No replacement of lost or stolen prescriptions
- Do not drink alcohol
- Do not use recreational drugs including marijuana
- Do not use with any other sedating drugs
- Proper disposal of excess drugs
- Description of behaviors that will result in taper and discontinuation of drug
- Consequences of failing to uphold the opioid agreement

Managing patient expectations are critical and are part of the informed consent process. Persons on COT for chronic noncancer pain typically report no more than a 20%–30% decrease in pain intensity (Chou et al., 2009). Improvement in function, sleep, mood, and social interactions are goals that are as important as the reduction in pain. A significant amount of time is needed to educate patients regarding the potential outcomes of chronic pain therapy.

Initiation of a new CS prescription should start as a *therapeutic trial* for a designated time period, for example, 1–2 months. The APRN and patient need to establish the criteria for a *successful trial* of a CS drug and what constitutes a lack of response. For example, improved functional level and improved sleep are realistic goals for a patient on opioids for chronic low back pain.

Differentiating between a failure to respond to opioid therapy versus inadequate opioid dosing can occasionally be quite challenging. For chronic noncancer pain, the opioid dose will be gradually escalated to achieve the desired effect. Responders will typically start to experience therapeutic benefits as the dose increases until an appropriate, stable opioid dose is achieved.

There is controversy regarding what constitutes a maximum therapeutic dose of COT for chronic noncancer pain, and no definition of what constitutes a "high" dose (Chou et al., 2009, p. 120). The American Pain Society/American Academy of Pain Medicine Guidelines report that 85% of all U.S. opioid prescriptions are in the range of 200 mg per day of morphine equivalent or less, and defines "high" opioid dose as over this amount (Chou et al., 2009). The Department of Veterans Affairs & Department of Defense Guidelines (2010) also define morphine equivalent of less than 200 mg per day as "low to moderate" dose range, and greater than 200 mg per day as "high" dose. Likewise, the recently updated Canadian Pain Society guidelines on COT describe doses over 200 mg of morphine equivalent per day as a "watchful dose" (Furlan, Reardon, Weppler, & National Opioid Use Guideline Group, 2010).

The Utah Department of Health guidelines state that "it seems reasonable to increase clinical vigilance at a daily dose that exceeds 120–200 mg of morphine equivalent per day" (Utah Department of Health, 2009, p. 15). The Washington State AMDG guidelines selected a dose of less than 120 mg per day morphine equivalent as the maximum acceptable dose for primary care providers who treat patients with chronic noncancer pain. These guidelines recommend specialist consultation if greater than 120 mg per day of morphine is required for COT.

If a therapeutic trial of opioids for chronic pain does not decrease pain and improve function, the drug should be tapered and discontinued. Consideration may be given to a trial of another opioid medication or other options for pain control such as use of anticonvulsants and antidepressants.

Writing monthly CS prescriptions is time-consuming and requires organization. The APRN should work with the practice's leadership to develop a plan that facilitates the care of patients who use CSs chronically to insure prescriptions are written in a timely manner, especially on holiday weekends and provider vacations. This will help prevent last minute urgent renewal requests and unpleasant or potentially dangerous symptoms related to acute withdrawal from opioids, benzodiazepines, or other CSs. Clinic policy should address issues such as opioid care agreements, UDT, and referral criteria.

Initiation of chronic opioid therapy for noncancer pain should be a deliberately planned therapy. Opioid therapy for chronic intermittent pain, for example, severe dysmenorrhea, needs to be regularly monitored to prevent unnecessary escalation of doses over time. Should an unintentional escalation of the opioid dose occur, consider initiating a formal pain management agreement.

Monitoring patients on long-term CS therapy

Patients on CSs should be followed regularly. Ongoing assessment of the 5 A's discussed above or use of a similar tool is needed. Occasional review of the diagnosis and repeat physical examination is needed at least once a year (Fishman, 2007). UDT, discussed above, is becoming more common in primary care. This is a controversial practice, and no established standards exist. Providers who utilize UDT usually administer the test randomly, once or twice a year. If concerning behaviors emerge, such as frequently missed appointments, requests for early refills, and behaviors suspicious for inappropriate use, the APRN should schedule more frequent visits, provide smaller quantities of CS prescriptions

(2-week supply instead of 30-day supply), and perform more frequent unannounced urine toxicology screens and pill counts.

Many authors describe the importance of having an *exit strategy* should it become necessary to stop the CS. A predetermined plan for discontinuing a CS will help the clinician in situations where the CS is clearly not working, expectations are not being met, or concerning behaviors are displayed. Strategies include scheduling a clinic visit to explain the problems, issues, and concerns to the patient. A plan may include tapering the CS over a period of time, initiation of other pain management strategies, clinician reassurance that the patient is not being abandoned, and specialist referral (Webster & Dove, 2007).

Any CS can be abused, and certain drugs have high street value and are at higher risk for diversion. These include oxycodone CR (OxyContin®), hydrocodone/acetaminophen (Vicodin®), hydromorphone (Dilaudid®), alprazolam (Xanax®), and methylphenidate (Ritalin®) (Webster & Dove, 2007). The APRN should limit or avoid prescribing these drugs to a patient evaluated to be at high risk for abuse or diversion. Other options for high-risk patients include avoiding short-acting opioids, use of methadone for pain, complementary and alternative therapies, over-the-counter medications, and biobehavioral approaches.

Distinguishing the abuser from the undermedicated patient

There is wide variability of responses to opioid pain medication. Undertreatment of pain and other disorders continues to be an ongoing problem. Patients whose pain is poorly managed because of provider discomfort with, or lack of expertise about, scheduled drugs is equally as unacceptable as prescribing inappropriately high doses (Weissman & Haddox, 1989). The term "opioidphobia" has been popularized to indicate clinicians fearful of prescribing opioids due to excessive concerns for disciplinary action or patients fearful of taking opioids due to excessive fears of "addiction."

People with mood disorders may present with behaviors that make it difficult to assess their need for, and response to, a CS. One challenge in prescribing CSs is to distinguish an abuser from the patient who needs a higher dose of drug for improved pain, anxiety, or hyperactivity management. How do you differentiate the two

---

Box 4.7 Behaviors related to predicting drug addiction

Aberrant behaviors less predictive of addiction
   Aggressive complaining about need for a higher dose
   Drug hoarding when symptoms are milder
   Requesting specific drugs
   Acquiring similar drugs from other medical sources
   Unsanctioned dose escalation once or twice
   Unapproved use of the drug to treat another symptom
   Reporting psychiatric drug-related effects not intended by the clinician
   Occasional impairment

Aberrant behaviors more predictive of addiction
   Selling prescription drugs
   Prescription forgery
   Stealing or "borrowing" drugs from another person
   Injecting oral formulations
   Obtaining prescription drugs from a nonmedical source
   Multiple episodes of prescription "loss"
   Concurrent abuse of related illicit drugs
   Multiple dose escalations despite warnings
   Repeated episodes of gross impairment or dishevelment

Source: Portenoy, 1996. Reprinted as adapted in Webster and Dove, 2007, with permission from Sunrise River Press.

---

groups? Even experienced providers may have difficulty. Certain behaviors are more typical of each group. Passik, Kirsh, Donaghy, and Portenoy (2006) conducted a study to review aberrant behaviors to determine which are less or more likely to indicate abuse of pain medications. The behaviors are displayed in Box 4.7.

Another useful tool to assess addictive behaviors is the "4 C's." Persons who are addicted to a medication demonstrate (1) impaired *control* over drug use, (2) *compulsive* use, (3) *continued* use despite obvious harm to self and others, and (4) drug *craving* (Smith & Passik, 2008, p. 427). This tool uses clear, straightforward language that can be used to educate patients or family members who fear becoming "addicted" to CSs.

Box 4.8 Common traits of the professional diverter

- Refuses or is reluctant to present identification
- Is "from out of town"
- Pays cash
- Requests controlled substances by telephone
- Schedules clinic visits for when the regular provider is unavailable
- Is in a hurry to leave the clinic
- Requests drugs by name
- Tries to control the interview
- Is well versed in clinical or street terminology
- Claims an allergy to nonsteroidal anti-inflammatory drugs, local anesthetics, or codeine
- Gives reasons why alternative pain treatments will not work
- Gives evasive answers
- Does not show up for follow-up visits
- Shows no interest in a diagnosis
- Claims no health insurance
- Has no regular provider
- Claims that previous medical records are unavailable
- Refuses physical examination
- Attempts to skip diagnostic tests
- Fakes naïveté about medications or medical condition
- Exaggerates or feigns symptoms
- Feigns psychiatric symptoms of anxiety, insomnia, or depression

Source: Reprinted from Webster and Dove, 2007, with permission from Sunrise River Press.

It is important to remain vigilant and identify drug seeking behavior that may cause the APRN to become the victim of a scam. A DEA (1999) resource, *Recognizing the Drug Abuser*, provides tools which will help the primary care practitioner to identify suspicious behaviors and prevent inappropriate prescribing. Common traits of the professional diverter are noted in Box 4.8. Tips to prevent forgery and diversion are included in Box 4.9.

Dealing with difficult situations

The "inherited patient," who transfers care from another provider while on chronic opioid or benzodiazepine therapy, may present a

---

Box 4.9 Prescribing tips to prevent forgery and diversion

- Keep blank prescription pads in a safe and secure place; do not leave them in exam rooms or areas accessible to patients; treat them like money.
- Use tamper-resistant prescription forms that cannot be photocopied.
- Use carbonless copies or make a copy of each CS prescription for the record. This can be used for comparison if the pharmacy contacts you with a question.
- Write out prescription strength and quantity:
  "oxycodone CR 10 (ten) mg q12 hours, dispense #20 (twenty)"
    (This prevents the number "10" from being changed to "40" or "70"; and the number "20" changed to "200.")
- Do not leave refill space blank, indicate "NR" for no refill.
- Write exact dates on prescription "To last from 4/1/2012 through 4/30/2012" or write "To last 30 days."

Source: PharmaCom Group Inc., 2007.

---

particular challenge for the APRN. Similar to an APRN's decision whether to continue an antihypertensive regimen, the APRN must decide whether to continue a CS regimen. The APRN may not concur with the patient's diagnosis or the type of controlled drug and/or dose prescribed. It may be difficult to determine the best approach to use (Gourlay & Heit, 2009). It is prudent to obtain records to review. The review should include evaluation of the problem that precipitated the need for the CS, and the patient's medication history including the CS used. If necessary, consult with the previous prescriber to gain an understanding of the history of the patient's management plan. If additional consultation is needed, an evaluation by a pain specialist could help the patient transition to a new approach to management of their CS.

The APRN is not obligated to prescribe CSs to a new patient. Many providers have a policy of *not* prescribing controlled drugs at the initial patient visit. Declining to prescribe does not represent patient abandonment. This is often a challenging and delicate situation. The patient may expect a CS prescription and may need it to prevent CS withdrawal. The APRN is well advised to create a plan to deal with these situations before they occur. Education and dialogue with the patient regarding concerns about the current regimen are essential. When the APRN chooses to alter the treatment plan, the changes should be clearly delineated in a written plan with a time line and the consequences of not following the plan.

Consultation

As with all other aspects of their practice, it is essential that APRNs understand the limits of their expertise and knowledge, and utilize consultants if needed. The management of patients who are long-term users of opioids or benzodiazepines can be complex and occasionally confusing. Discussing a case with a trusted colleague can provide perspective. The VA/DoD Guidelines on Opioid Therapy for chronic pain (2010) provide helpful criteria for patient referral to a pain medicine specialist or a behavioral health specialist. Many, if not most, pain specialists will assess the patient and make recommendations, but will not assume responsibility for prescribing opioids on a chronic basis.

The APRN is advised to work closely with the consultant to develop a pharmacological treatment plan that is congruent with what is feasible within the primary care environment. Similarly, some psychiatrists will provide consultation on pharmacological management of psychiatric illness, but will not prescribe CSs on an ongoing basis.

SUMMARY

As APRNs have gained broader prescriptive authority, understanding the complex issues related to prescribing CSs have become essential. This chapter has addressed methods to prescribe CSs safely, while remaining aware of potential inappropriate use. The APRN must approach CS prescribing with vigilance and caution, without becoming unduly fearful or "opioidphobic."

Recently published professional guidelines provide excellent direction to the clinician prescribing opioids for chronic pain. These strategies may be applied to other categories of CSs. By utilizing "Universal Precautions in Pain Medicine" (Gourlay et al., 2005), including written treatment agreement plans, the astute APRN will provide a consistent approach to all patients receiving opioids or other CSs. This approach will help avoid inappropriate prescribing, provide strategies to deal with unexpected findings, and provide reassurance that the plan of care is within generally accepted standards. Although prescribing CSs can be complex and time-consuming, these drugs have the ability to significantly improve the quality of life for people with pain, anxiety, or other disorders. Controlled substances are not to be feared or avoided, simply used judiciously.

REFERENCES

Agency Medical Directors Group (AMDG). (2010). Interagency guideline on opioid dosing for chronic non-cancer pain: An educational aid to improve care and safety with opioid therapy. Retrieved from http://www.agencymeddirectors.wa.gov/Files/OpioidGdline.pdf

American Academy of Pain Medicine. (2010). AAPMedicine applauds the inclusion of pain care in new healthcare reform. Retrieved from http://www.painmed.org/files/aapm-applauds-inclusion-of-pain-care-in-new-healthcare-reform.pdf

American Academy of Pain Medicine, American Pain Society, & American Society of Addiction Medicine. (2001). Consensus document from the American Academy of Pain Medicine, the American Pain Society, and the American Society of Addiction Medicine on definitions related to the use of opioids for the treatment of pain. Retrieved from http://www.pcssmethadone.org/pcss/documents2/ASAM_DefinitionsRelatedToUseOpioidsPain.pdf

American Geriatrics Society Panel on Pharmacological Management of Persistent Pain in Older Persons. (2009). Pharmacological management of persistent pain in older persons. *Journal of the American Geriatrics Society*, *57*(8), 1331–1346.

Boswell, M. V., & Giordano, J. (2009). Reflection, analysis and change: The decade of pain control and research and its lessons for the future of pain management. *Pain Physician*, *12*(2), 923–928.

Bramness, J. G., Furu, K., & Engeland, A. (2007). Carisoprodol use and abuse in Norway. A pharmacoepidemiological study. *British Journal Clinical Pharmacology*, *64*(2), 210–218.

Bramness, J. G., & Skurtveit, S. (2008). Carisoprodol should be taken off the market. *Southern Medical Journal*, *101*(10), 1074–1075.

Carlozzi, A. F., Fornari, F. A., Siwicki, D. M., Barkin, R., Nafziger, A. N., Woodcock, M., . . . Aronoff, G. (2008). Urine drug monitoring: Opioids. North Kingstown, RI: Dominion Diagnostics. Retrieved from http://www.painmedicinenews.com/download/PG0818_WM.pdf

Chou, R. (2010). What we still don't know about treating chronic noncancer pain with opioids. *Canadian Medical Association Journal, 182*(9), 881–882.

Chou, R., Fanciullo, G. J., Fine, P. G., Adler, J. A., Ballantyne, J. C., Davies, P., . . . Miaskowski, C. (2009). Clinical guidelines for the use of chronic opioid therapy in chronic noncancer pain. *The Journal of Pain, 10*(2), 113–130.

Ciraulo, D. M., & Ciraulo, D. A. (2008). Benzodiazepines. In H. S. Smith, & S. D. Passik (Eds.), *Pain and chemical dependency* (pp. 137–144). New York: Oxford University Press.

Cleeland, C. S., & Ryan, K. M. (1994). Pain assessment: Global use of the brief pain inventory. *Annals of the Academy of Medicine, Singapore, 23*(2), 129–138.

Comer, S. D., & Ashworth, J. B. (2008). The growth of prescription opioid abuse. In H. S. Smith, & S. D. Passik (Eds.), *Pain and chemical dependency* (pp. 19–23). New York: Oxford University Press.

Department of Veterans Affairs & Department of Defense. (2010). VA/DoD clinical practice guideline for management of opioid therapy for chronic pain. Retrieved from http://www.healthquality.va.gov/cot/cot_310_sum.pdf

Drug Abuse Warning Network (DAWN). (2011). Drug abuse warning network, 2008: national estimates of drug-related emergency department visits. Retrieved from http://www.oas.samhsa.gov/DAWN/2K8/ED/DAWN2k8ED.pdf

Drug Enforcement Administration. (1999). Don't be scammed by a drug abuser. Retrieved from https://www.deadiversion.usdoj.gov/pubs/brochures/drugabuser.htm

Drug Enforcement Administration. (2009). Drugs and chemicals of concern: Tramadol. Office of Diversion Control. Retrieved from http://www.deadiversion.usdoj.gov/drugs_concern/tramadol.pdf

Federation of State Medical Boards. (2004). Model policy for the use of controlled substances for the treatment of pain. Retrieved from http://www.fsmb.org/pdf/2004_grpol_Controlled_ Substances.pdf

Federation of State Medical Boards. (2010). Resources for pharmacovigilance and pain management. Retrieved from http://www. fsmb.org/PAIN/resource.html

Fishman, S. M. (2007). *Responsible opioid prescribing: A physician's guide*. Washington, DC: Waterford Life Science.

Food and Drug Administration. (2010). Ultram (tramadol hydrochloride), Ultracet (tramadol hydrochloride/acetaminophen): Label change. Retrieved from http://www.fda.gov/Safety/ MedWatch/SafetyInformation/SafetyAlertsforHumanMedical Products/ucm213264.htm

Furlan, A. D., Reardon, R., Weppler, C., & National Opioid Use Guideline Group. (2010). Opioids for chronic noncancer pain: A new Canadian practice guideline. *Canadian Medical Association Journal, 182*(9), 923–930.

Geriatrics and Extended Care Strategic Healthcare Group. (2000). Take 5. Pain: The 5th vital sign. Veterans Health Administration. Retrieved from http://www1.va.gov/PAINMANAGEMENT/ docs/TOOLKIT.pdf

Gourlay, D. L., & Heit, H. A. (2006). Universal precautions: A matter of mutual trust and responsibility. *Pain Medicine, 7*(2), 210–211.

Gourlay, D. L. & Heit, H. A. (2009). Universal precautions revisited: managing the inherited pain patient. *Pain Medicine, 10*(Suppl 2), S115–S123.

Gourlay, D. L., Heit, H. A., & Almahrezi, A. (2005). Universal precautions in pain medicine: A rational approach to the treatment of chronic pain. *Pain Medicine, 6*(2), 107–112.

Institute of Medicine. (2011). Relieving pain in America: A blueprint for transforming prevention, care, education, and research. Retrieved from www.iom.edu/reports/2011/Relieving-Pain-in_America-A-Blueprint-for-Transforming-Prevention-Care-Education-Research.aspx

The Joint Commission. (2011). Facts about pain management. Retrieved from http://www.jointcommission.org/assets/1/18/ Pain_Management.pdf

Katz, N. P., Sherburne, S., Beach, M., Rose, R. J., Vielguth, J., Bradley, J., & Fanciullo, G. J. (2003). Behavioral monitoring and urine toxicology testing in patients receiving long-term opioid therapy. *Anesthesia & Analgesia*, 97(4), 1097–1102.

The Management of Opioid Therapy for Chronic Pain Working Group. (2010). VA/DoD clinical practice guideline for management of opioid therapy for chronic pain. Retrieved from http://www.va.gov/PAINMANAGEMENT/docs/CPG_opioidtherapy_fulltext.pdf

Nabati, L., & Abrahm, J. (2008). The palliative care patient. In H. S. Smith, & S. D. Passik (Eds.), *Pain and chemical dependency* (pp. 321–328). New York: Oxford University Press.

National Drug Intelligence Center. (2009). National prescription drug threat assessment. Retrieved from http://www.justice.gov/ndic/pubs33/33775/index.htm

Pain & Policy Studies Group. (2008). Achieving balance in state pain policy: A report card (4th ed.). Retrieved from http://www.painpolicy.wisc.edu/Achieving_Balance/PRC2008.pdf

Passik, S. D., & Kirsh, K. L. (2008). Chemical coping: The clinical middle ground. In H. S. Smith, & S. D. Passik (Eds.), *Pain and chemical dependency* (pp. 299–302). New York: Oxford University Press.

Passik, S. D., Kirsh, K. L., Donaghy, K. B., & Portenoy, R. S. (2006). Pain and aberrant drug-related behaviors in medically ill patients with and without histories of substance abuse. *Clinical Journal of Pain*, 22(2), 173–181.

PharmaCom Group Inc. (2007). *Tips, photographs, & explanations: A practical guide for prescribing controlled substances* (1st ed.). Stamford, CT: Alpharma Pharmaceuticals.

Portenoy, R. K. (1996). Opioid therapy for chronic nonmalignant pain: A review of the critical issues. *Journal of Pain and Symptom Management*, 11(4), 203–217.

Reeves, R. R., & Burke, R. S. (2010). Carisoprodol: Abuse potential and withdrawal syndrome. *Current Drug Abuse Review*, 3(1), 33–38.

Savage, S. R. (2008). The language of pain and addiction. In H. S. Smith, & S. D. Passik (Eds.), *Pain and chemical dependency* (pp. 9–10). New York: Oxford University Press.

Schutte-Rodin, S., Broch, L., Buysse, D., Dorsey, C., & Sateia, M. (2008). Clinical guideline for the evaluation and management of chronic insomnia in adults. *Journal of Clinical Sleep Medicine*, 4(5), 487–504.

Smith, H. S., & Passik, S. D. (Eds.). (2008). *Pain and chemical dependency*. New York: Oxford University Press.

Stedman, T. L. (2006). *Stedman's medical dictionary*. Philadelphia: Lippincott Williams & Wilkins.

Suddath, C. (2009). The war on drugs. *Time*. Retrieved from http://www.time.com/time/world/article/0,8599,1887488,00.html

Utah Department of Health. (2009). Utah clinical guidelines on prescribing opioids for pain. Retrieved from http://health.utah.gov/prescription/pdf/guidelines/final.04.09opioidGuidlines.pdf

Webster, L. R., & Dove, B. (2007). *Avoiding opioid abuse while managing pain: A guide for practitioners*. North Branch, MN: Sunrise River Press.

Weissman, D. E., & Haddox, J. D. (1989). Opioid pseudoaddiction: An iatrogenic syndrome. *Pain*, 36(3), 363–366.

Managing Difficult Patient Situations

5

Donna Poole, Marie Annette Brown, and Louise Kaplan

Chapter 5 coaches advanced practice registered nurses (APRNs) to deal with difficult and often complex clinical situations that are inherent in professional practice interactions. The basic tenet is that these are not "problem patients," but situations for which the APRN needs more knowledge, skill, and insight from self-reflection. Information to enhance understanding of why these difficult situations develop and how they can impact patient-centered care is presented. Specific strategies to identify difficult situations, respond to them appropriately, and build competence as a supportive and courageous APRN prescriber are discussed.

A hallmark of advanced practice registered nurse (APRN) practice is establishing caring, supportive relationships with patients in order to "make a difference" in patients' lives. Many APRNs attribute their satisfaction with their work and longevity in the role to these rewarding or inspiring relationships with patients (Brown & Draye, 2003). At the same time, interactions with patients can be a source of significant stress. APRNs are often faced with clinical situations that are prompted by stressful patient interactions that they find difficult or for which they feel ill prepared. There is usually little education aimed at increasing knowledge and skills to assist APRNs to manage these particular types of clinical situations.

The Advanced Practice Registered Nurse as a Prescriber, First Edition. Marie Annette Brown, Louise Kaplan.
© 2012 John Wiley & Sons, Ltd. Published 2012 by John Wiley & Sons, Ltd.

Certain patient behaviors can be particularly uncomfortable for many clinicians. The insightful discussion by Miksanek (2008) offers expert guidance and encouragement to all providers. He urges clinicians to first acknowledge their feelings about these patient situations in order to transform frustration into hope. His article "On Caring for 'Difficult' Patients," offers a provocative introduction about this dilemma.

> Let's be blunt. It's hard to care for difficult patients. It's sometimes impossible to actually like them. This species of sick individuals tends to strain time, patience and resources. They often generate a cascade of phone calls. They sometimes demand a heap of medically unnecessary tests. They occasionally refuse recommended treatment. Many have unreasonable expectations. Some whine and gripe incessantly. A few threaten to sue. Almost all of them need at least thirty minutes—and want sixty minutes—of face time. . . . In their own unique ways, they make my professional life tricky. Even in my private life, they invade my thoughts—with disappointment, irritation and worry. (p. 1422)

Healthcare providers may react and intensify the challenging interpersonal situations rather than respond in a thoughtful and informed manner to prevent escalation of the current problem. Common difficult situations may include:

- patients who are or appear to be drug seeking
- patients who act out their anger
- patients who act arrogant and/or entitled
- patients who violate boundaries
- patients who request inappropriate or unnecessary care (e.g., antibiotics for the common cold)
- patients who choose not to adopt treatment recommendations
- patients who do not improve according to expectations.

The word *patient* originally meant "one who suffers" and is derived from the Latin word *patiens*, meaning "I am suffering" (*Merriam-Webster Dictionary*, 2011). The practitioner may also suffer in common difficult situations with feelings of psychological distress or a sense of failure. When a practitioner feels frustrated, uncertain, angry, manipulated, or controlled, the patient may be labeled a "problem patient." While many providers and publications assume that the patient is a difficult person with whom to interact, there are also provider and healthcare system factors that contribute to the situations (Haas, Leiser, Magill, & Sanyer, 2005). Gender may also be a significant influence on one's interaction style, particularly with assertiveness and self-advocacy. Amanatullah and Morris (2010) hypothesize that women are "savvy impression managers" and, so as not to be perceived as violating gender roles, avoid self-advocacy. However, in their study, they did find that advocacy on behalf of others is quite consistent with community expectations.

One estimate is that 5%–10% of patients in a typical primary-care practice are considered difficult to deal with by their providers (Keaveney, 2004). Despite the pervasiveness of this issue, research in this area is limited across the health professions (Koekkoek, Meijel, & Hutschemaekers, 2006). Current research and evidence-based approaches to this topic are particularly sparse.

A 2006 literature review of articles published between 1979 and 2004 focusing on the "difficult patient" noted that the majority of the data was published before 1991 (Koekkoek et al., 2006). Analysis of this information about difficult patient behaviors fell into four categories: the withdrawn and hard to reach, the demanding and claiming, the attention seeking and manipulative, and the aggressive and dangerous. Additionally, they found that while there were no studies dealing solely with the role of the professional, there were personality traits in professionals that tended to increase the risk of difficult relationships with patients. These traits include: a strong wish to cure; a great need to care, trouble with accepting defeat, and a confrontational and blaming attitude. Further evidence is needed to better understand personal characteristics such as competitiveness, propensity for "power struggles," or the need to "be right" that may require clinicians to become more engaged in self-reflection and professional growth.

Many health professionals struggle with challenging patient interactions and attempt to keep patients who make them uncomfortable out of their practice. Some might be successful at this; however, there are ethical implications if care is refused. How does the APRN resolve conflicts between duties to oneself and duties to the patient? Patients generally seek consultation because they are suffering. It is the responsibility of the practitioner to help patients address their health needs. It is also the responsibility of the practitioner to develop expertise in handling conflicts and disagreements that arise in professional interactions. Lack of expertise with difficult clinical situations can prompt clinicians to struggle with feelings of inadequacy, leading them to reject or avoid patients (Jones, 2004).

There are numerous approaches a practitioner can use to prepare to handle the most common difficult situations. This may also increase the practitioner's comfort and competence in managing difficult situations, decrease work stress, and increase job satisfaction. This chapter provides a conceptual framework and strategies for managing some of the most common difficulties that APRNs may face in their relationships with patients.

COUNTERTRANSFERENCE

Although there is little research related to dealing with difficult patient situations, patients are generally considered "difficult" because of the special intensity of feelings, or countertransference (Roberts & Dyer, 2003). Countertransference is a concept that may be unfamiliar to most APRNs outside the psychiatric/mental health specialty. However, its basic tenets apply to our daily interactions with both patients and colleagues and are particularly relevant in the prescriber role. It can be used to move the clinician's focus from "difficult patients" to the complexity of human relationships.

Countertransference is unconscious feelings that may be inappropriate to the content and context of the relationship (Stuart, 2009). When they are driving the professional relationship, the manifestations can be negative and conflict ridden. A hallmark of countertransference is feelings toward patients of an increased intensity. The expression of countertransference can occur in a variety of ways ranging from benign to serious. Frequent countertransference reactions include: anger, impatience, resentment (Pearson, 2001), intense anxiety, disgust, hostility in response to resistance from the patient (Stuart, 2009), over- or underinvolvement with patients, physical symptoms, and negative perceptions of patients. Other examples of countertransference include:

"• difficulty empathizing with the patient concerning certain problem areas
• feelings of anger or impatience because of the patient's unwillingness to change

- recurrent anxiety, unease, or guilt related to the patient
- a tendency to focus on only one aspect or way of looking at information provided by the patient
- experiences strong emotional reactions
- finds it necessary to talk to someone about the patient
- allows violations of boundaries to occur
- engages in behaviors that cannot be justified as therapeutic
- experiences a desire to please or avoid
- is preoccupied with another and/or engages in power struggles" (Stuart, 2009, p. 40).

When countertransference leads to over- or under-involvement with patients, it may lead to a loss of boundaries and a career-ending encounter. Over-involvement may be as simple as giving a patient something that one would not ordinarily give to others, such as a gift, excessive time, or a special service. Providing a patient with unwarranted prescriptions serves as another key example. An extreme loss of boundaries may result in serious ethical violations such as sexual contact with patients. Clinicians experiencing difficult personal situations such as divorce or separation from a partner or death of a family member may be particularly vulnerable to boundary issues. While feelings of attraction to a patient may occur, acting on this attraction is unacceptable.

Under-involvement with patients may manifest as avoidance or impersonalization. Referring to patients by their illness or characteristics is one way of creating an impersonal distance, for example, the "headache" patient. Stronger feelings of disdain or aversion toward a patient may lead to more serious avoidance or neglect resulting in harm to the patient (see Box 5.1).

As with most emotional reactions or stress triggers, physical symptoms or bodily reactions may manifest as part of counter-transference. APRNs can be particularly mindful of their own characteristic physical reactions to stress, such as increased heart or respiration rate, chest tightness, sweating, jaw clenching, tightening neck or abdominal muscles, and gastrointestinal distress. For example, these symptoms may be triggered when an APRN declines a patient's request for antibiotics for a viral infection and a patient insists that is the only thing that has helped in the past.

Box 5.1 Case example: negligence

A male patient was a frequent visitor to a busy primary care practice. He typically presented with a long list of concerns and questions which he reviewed in detail with the APRN. Over time, the clinic more narrowly defined "productivity" expectations by the number of patients seen. In response, the APRN became increasingly annoyed, impatient, and concerned about the time demands from this particular patient and worried about a poor performance evaluation. He began to view this patient as a "crock." As a consequence, over the years, he did not pay attention to rising prostate-specific antigen (PSA) levels, and the patient was eventually diagnosed with metastatic prostate cancer. In addition to the patient's suffering, the APRN was successfully sued for negligence.

Monitoring one's own individual physical responses may often provide a window into countertransference.

The way in which APRNs experience and learn to handle countertransference can have profound effects on their relationships with patients. APRNs that pay little attention to countertransference may unintentionally create difficulties in their clinical practice. Lack of awareness of countertransference may also trigger aggression in a patient. An angry and hostile response to an angry or hostile patient may escalate the situation. Anger or sarcasm expressed during a discussion about medication options is rarely a helpful approach to facilitating a patient's self-care. Awareness of countertransference can lead to a deeper and more meaningful understanding of the patient. For example, symptoms of depression may occur when working with a depressed patient (Anderson, Hoop, & Roberts, 2009).

When the APRN experiences these reactions during a patient interaction, it is critical to address them. Similarly, the labeling of patients may be a "red flag" to the presence of countertransference. For example, two commonly used labels among healthcare professionals referring to a patient are "noncompliant" or "drug seeking." Some may use even more pejorative terms. Because these terms often reflect feelings of powerlessness, the clinician may try even harder to control the patient, leading to further struggle. "Control is a concept of 'power over' whereas competence can be seen as 'power to'. . . . [APRNs] need to minimize the former and maximize the latter" (Stuart, 2009, p. 41).

Self-reflection is an important skill to help APRNs remain vigilant about their behavior and address areas of concern. It can also be useful for APRNs to focus on their emotional well-being to ascertain if a "need to be liked" and accepted by patients contributes to a conflict-avoidant approach to patient interactions. When APRNs are alert to cues, they may become aware of their emotions, develop insight, improve the quality of patient care, and prevent damage to professional relationships (O'Kelly, 1998).

APRNs are also encouraged to engage in honest self-reflection by asking: "Is the service or object being provided something that could be revealed to others?" and "Would I feel proud or ashamed if colleagues and patients were aware of this service or medication prescribed?" With the complexity of current practice, there is an even greater need for focused self-questioning as part of an ongoing dialogue within oneself and with colleagues.

More than half a century ago, Peplau (1951) identified that for a nurse to assist patients to meet their needs, the nurse must be aware of his or her own needs. These very human needs are part of each individual's collective life experience and may arise in situations where the APRN feels particularly vulnerable. They are, however, an expected dimension of lifelong learning and professional growth. Driscoll and Teh (2001) highlight essential antecedents that could help APRNs to fulfill a commitment to reflective practice. The antecedents of reflective practice can be seen in Box 5.2. Self-reflection is essential for APRNs who must grapple with multiple issues that are part of the prescribing role. Reflective practice is not only considered an essential skill but part of the basic foundation and "worldview" of APRNs. "Reflective practice is an active and deliberate process of critically examining practice where an individual is challenged and enabled to undertake the process of self-enquiry to empower the practitioner to realize desirable and effective practice within a reflexive spiral of personal transformation" (Duffy, 2007, p. 1405).

In summary, countertransference may manifest through the level of involvement of the APRN with the patient, physical symptoms, and in the APRN's positive and negative descriptions of the patient. Countertransference can be regarded as normal or inevitable and if recognized can be used to improve the well-being of the patient and provide depth to the APRN's practice expertise.

Box 5.2 Antecedents of reflective practice

- A willingness to learn from what happens in practice
- Being open enough to share elements of practice with other people
- Being aware of the conditions necessary for reflection to occur
- A belief that it is possible to change as a practitioner
- The ability to describe in detail before analyzing practice problems
- Recognizing the consequences of reflection
- The ability to articulate what happens in practice
- A belief that there is no end point in learning about practice
- Not being defensive about what other people notice about one's practice
- Being courageous enough to act on reflection
- Working out schemes to personally action what has been learned
- Being honest
- Being motivated enough to "replay" aspects of clinical practice [or review patient interactions to assess for improvement]
- Knowledge for clinical practice can emerge from within, as well outside clinical practice

Source: Reprinted from Duffy (2007), with permission from the *British Journal of Nursing*.

ETHICAL CONSIDERATIONS WHEN DEALING WITH DIFFICULT SITUATIONS

National polls repeatedly identify nurses as the public's most trusted profession (Jones, 2010). The professional ethics of APRNs have contributed to the public's esteem. Nonetheless, the complexity of prescribing and factors such as direct-to-consumer advertising of medication may create difficult clinical situations between APRNs and patients. When this occurs, the Code of Ethics for Nurses with Interpretive Statements (American Nurses Association, 2001) can provide guidance.

The first official Code of Ethics for Nurses was adopted by the American Nurses Association in 1950 with the current version adopted in 2001. Of the nine provisions, the first and the fifth provisions are most applicable to dealing with difficult situations.

Provision 1: The Nurse, in all professional relationships, practices with compassion and respect for the inherent dignity, worth, and uniqueness of every individual, unrestricted by considerations of social or economic status, personal attributes, or the nature of health problems.

Provisions 5: The Nurse owes the same duties to self as to others, including the responsibility to preserve integrity and safety, to maintain competence, and to continue personal and professional growth.

Provision 1 represents the core values and responsibilities of the profession. This ethic translates into respect for all persons and includes patients who are difficult or bring challenges to the relationship that may lead to feelings of anxiety or discomfort. This spectrum ranges from patients who request unnecessary medications to patients who are substance abusers.

Provision 5 includes wholeness of character, identity, and integrity (Fowler, 2000). Respect for oneself is implied if not explicit. This provision may be interpreted to highlight that the APRN is responsible for his or her own feelings and the management of self. The APRN also has a responsibility to place the well-being of all patients in the forefront. This responsibility includes patients who engage in behaviors that do not serve them well such as the intentional failure to provide complete and accurate information or devious actions in order to meet a need. These behaviors are common among patients who are known or are suspected to abuse controlled substances.

Similarly, the ethical code of the American Society of Pain Management Nurses reflects the commitment to providing care to individuals who are substance abusers. The "…principles of beneficence (the duty to benefit another) and justice (the equal or comparative treatment of individuals) oblige healthcare professionals to manage pain and provide humane care to all patients, including those patients known or suspected to have addictive disease" (American Society for Pain Management Nursing [ASPMN], 2011).

DIFFICULT SITUATIONS IN WHICH SUBSTANCE ABUSE IS SUSPECTED

The problem of prescription substance abuse

The National Institute on Drug Abuse (NIDA) reports that prescription drug abuse is a serious and growing public health problem in the United States (NIDA, 2011). It estimates that approximately 20% of the U.S. population will use prescription drugs for nonmedical purposes in their lifetime. One study demonstrated that 2.5% of the population used prescription drugs for nonmedical reasons in 2008 (O'Malley, 2010).

As a result of the growing problem of prescription drug abuse, APRNs are sometimes in a position to manage difficult clinical situations when there is suspected abuse of controlled substances. Abuse of drugs can present in many forms (Substance Abuse and Mental Health Services Administration [SAMHSA], 2008). Some patients establish care when they are already dependent upon a controlled substance. Other patients may develop substance abuse patterns over time in an attempt to self-medicate for physical or emotional health problems (Wilford, 1990). Some patients may seek to obtain medications for a family member or friend or to sell the drug, which is known as diversion (Childress, 2004).

The Substance Abuse and Mental Health Services Administration reports that pain relievers, tranquilizers, stimulants, and sedatives are the controlled substances most commonly used for nonmedical purposes. Each class of medications has a specific effect on brain neurotransmitters. All appear to trigger dopamine release of the "reward pathway" causing an altered state of consciousness seen as desirable by some individuals (Longo, Parran, Johnson, & Kinsey, 2000).

APRNs may have concerns that prescribing controlled substances could contribute to problems of abuse, addiction, and dependence. Preventing or reducing prescription drug abuse is an important part of providing care to patients. However, avoiding controlled substances when they are needed because of that fear can affect the quality of care delivered by APRNs. To successfully navigate between the dichotomy of relieving suffering and contributing to harm, it is important for the prescriber to develop the expertise to identify a drug abuser.

Definitions

The term that is most frequently used to describe aberrant drug behavior in professional discussions and literature is "drug seeking." The term is poorly defined and is often used pejoratively. It may be applied to patients considered difficult or who challenge the APRN in order to control the type or amount of controlled substance prescribed. The ASPMN recommended that terms such as "drug seeking" not be used as they create stigma, prejudice, bias, and barriers to care (ASPMN, 2011). In one study, over 80% of nurses agreed that the term "drug seeking" had a negative meaning; 50% admitted using the term when talking about patients, but over 90% stated they did not use the term in charting. The study's authors described the stigmatizing effect of the term and suggest instead the phrase "concern-raising behaviors" so as not to prejudge patients (McCaffery, Grimm, Pasero, Ferrell, & Uman, 2005).

Practitioners are often unclear about the distinctions among the terms of addiction, dependence, and tolerance, and use them incorrectly (see Chapter 4 for a more detailed discussion). Furthermore, patients who are reluctant to use specific controlled substances typically explain that they fear "addiction" to a specific medication. Because this is an inappropriate use of the word addiction, it can be an excellent "teachable moment" for APRNs to help patients understand how medications were developed for specific symptoms. At the same time, it is important to educate patients not suspected of inappropriate medication use about a medication's abuse potential. The ultimate goal of healthcare providers is to use judicious prescribing practices and avoid becoming the agent of iatrogenic dependence. Patients who ask for additional medication and may be suspected of "drug seeking" could in fact have "pseudoaddiction," which results from undertreatment of chronic pain (Fisher, 2004). While tolerance, dependence, and addiction are separate conditions, they can all exist in the same person. The terms as defined by ASPMN can be found in Box 5.3.

Identifying concern-raising behaviors

Open, trusting relationships with patients are an important practice goal for APRNs. It is essential, however, to avoid blind trust. In situations that have potential for abuse or misuse, APRNs must be alert to the possibility of purposeful misinformation and have an increased index of suspicion, as a patient may feign symptoms to achieve a goal.

Practitioners may say they use intuition to make decisions about possible abuse or misuse. A better understanding of intuition has helped nurses realize the systematic data and clinical expertise

---

Box 5.3 Definitions from the American Society for Pain Management Nursing

Addiction: A chronic, relapsing, treatable disease of the brain characterized by craving, dysfunctional behaviors, and an inability to control impulses regarding consumption of a substance or substances with compulsive use despite harmful consequences.

Physical dependence: An expected physiological response to a number of drug classes (such as opioids and benzodiazepines) that produces a drug class-specific withdrawal/abstinence syndrome (with drug class-specific symptoms) that is precipitated by abrupt cessation, rapid dose reduction, decreasing blood level of the drug, and/or administration of an antagonist.

Tolerance: A state of adaptation in which exposure to a drug induces changes that result in a diminution of one or more of the drug's effects over time.

Pseudoaddiction: An iatrogenic syndrome associated with the undertreatment of pain; characterized by various problematic behaviors that appear abuse-like. Pseudoaddiction can be distinguished from true addiction in that the behaviors resolve when pain is effectively treated.

Source: Reprinted with permission from the American Society for Pain Management Nursing. For the most up-to-date definitions, visit http://www.aspmn.org/.

---

that serves as the basis for intuition. Benner and Tanner (1987) define intuition as "understanding without a rationale" (p. 23), based on background understanding and skilled clinical observation. Pattern recognition occurs from the wisdom embedded in experience that is used as data against which the current situation is compared. Intuition is a legitimate and essential aspect of clinical judgment that is learned from experience. Consequently, it is often more difficult for inexperienced practitioners to use intuition or pattern recognition from previous experience to identify situations where abuse could or does occur.

There are a number of generally accepted warning signs in the identification of patients who may have concern-raising behaviors or medication use patterns. A patient's request for a specific drug by name regardless of diagnosis is one concern-raising behavior

(Robbins, 2007). Often the claim will be made that only one or two medications are effective and that other treatments do not work (Childress, 2004; Drug Enforcement Administration, 1999; Roscoe, 2004). They may be hesitant to try a more appropriate drug or resist other forms of therapy, such as physical therapy for pain or psychotherapy for anxiety. Claims of "allergy" to a more appropriate drug are also common. Brand name drugs have greater street value because they are more easily recognized as genuine (Longo et al., 2000; Robbins, 2007). As a consequence, complaints of allergies to generics pose a concern and should be explored thoroughly particularly when prescribing a controlled substance. It is important to note, however, that there are legitimate situations when a patient responds better to a brand name than a generic medication.

Drug abusers may show no interest in their diagnosis. The relationship of a drug abuser to their drug is stronger than any relationship they have with the provider or with the diagnosis (Longo et al., 2000). The history provided may also be vague or incomplete. A recommendation to refer them to a specialist for consultation or for diagnostic testing may be met with outright refusal, or they may fail to follow through with a workup to determine the diagnosis (Childress, 2004; Wilford, 1990). Refusal to be appropriately evaluated provides the basis for the APRN to refuse treatment with controlled substances.

Patients who feign physical symptoms are likely to be seeking opioids (Drug Enforcement Administration, 1999). Clues for detecting drug-seeking behavior can be the declaration of unusual symptoms that are physiologically implausible. In some instances, patients present with symptoms that are vague and difficult to clearly identify. Conversely, others report symptoms that mirror a professional textbook description (Robbins, 2007). Common presenting complaints for opioids abusers include kidney stones, abdominal or back pain, toothache, or migraine headaches (Drug Enforcement Administration, 1999). Clearly, most patients who present with pain-related conditions are not drug abusers. However, some healthcare professionals have difficulty differentiating those who present with legitimate complaints from those who do not. The practitioner must carefully assess and evaluate each situation using the approach recommended in Chapter 4.

Patients who feign psychological symptoms are likely to be seeking stimulants or benzodiazepines (Drug Enforcement Administration, 1999). They may present as self-diagnosed with attention deficit hyperactivity disorder (ADHD) or with complaints of anxiety, insomnia, fatigue, depression, or suicidality. This creates a dilemma for the practitioner in sorting through which of these complaints may be genuine and which may be bogus. As with the patient who feigns physical symptoms, the practitioner needs to assess and evaluate the patient with psychological symptoms using the approach recommended in Chapter 4.

In the author's experience, patients who have a known history of recreational stimulant abuse or dependence may justify their drug abuse by attributing it to a health problem that prompted self-medication through substances such as cocaine or methamphetamine. Some factors may assist APRNs as they differentiate between patients with and without concern-raising behaviors. Determine if the patient is willing to try treatment with a different medication than is being requested and if previous records support a diagnosis of a specific health problem.

Patients may threaten suicide if not provided with their medication of choice. These threats must be taken seriously and appropriately assessed. However, the threat clearly is an inappropriate rationale to prompt the APRN to acquiesce to a patient's request.

Patient ploys

Patients can use different ploys in an attempt to obtain medications. A patient who is overly flattering, especially on the first visit, may intend to manipulate the APRN to provide the requested medication (Roscoe, 2004). Conversely, patients may be extremely assertive and demanding because they understand a provider's desire to avoid confrontation. Patients sometimes attempt to elicit sympathy or guilt. Sympathy is usually engendered by sad personal stories. Guilt may be induced by accusing the practitioner of refusing the only medication that has ever been helpful to relieve suffering in the past. Established patients may also accuse practitioners of "causing them" to be dependent upon a medication as a method of evoking guilt (Drug Enforcement Administration, 1999). (See Box 5.4.)

Patients have also been known to offer bribes or pressure the APRN to provide a specific medication. A patient may also mention

---

Box 5.4 Case example: miscommunication despite use of a medication agreement

A 41-year-old female reported her long-time APRN to the state board of nursing for not providing appropriate consent in the beginning of treatment with a benzodiazepine. The patient decided to stop her medications without consulting the APRN and went through withdrawal symptoms, for which she was also not prepared. The records showed that the APRN had offered to provide medication treatment when she learned of the withdrawal. There was also a benzodiazepine management agreement in place that outlined the risk for tolerance and dependence. Following investigation by the state board, the charges were dismissed as "no violation" upon the strength of the APRNs documentation. However, the APRN spent several months anxious and stressed while waiting for the outcome of the investigation, and the relationship with the patient was irrevocably damaged.

---

an important person they purport to know who will negatively impact the practice if the APRN does not accede to their wishes. Patients who are "studying" the practitioner closely may also be searching for manipulative strategies appropriate to the current environment (Wilford, 1990).

The APRN is advised to pay attention to medication requests from a transient patient (Drug Enforcement Administration, 1999; Wilford, 1990). This may be someone from out of town with lost or stolen medications who presents with intense pain and a sense of urgency. Verification of the names and phone numbers of past or current prescribers and pharmacies may be helpful, as well as a complete review of past medical records (Roscoe, 2004). Often, national chain pharmacies are able to provide a patient's medication history, and many states track prescriptions for Medicaid patients.

Prescription monitoring programs (PMPs) for controlled substances are effective tools to identify and prevent drug diversion at the patient, prescriber, and pharmacy levels. As of 2011, thirty-four states have systems that are operating and another nine have legislation authorizing implementation of a program. PMPs collect and analyze electronically transmitted data from pharmacies and dispensing providers. Depending on state law, data may be available to prescribers, pharmacists, pharmacies, law enforcement, licensing boards, patients, agencies such as Medicaid or Medicare, and to researchers as de-identified data. States monitor some or all schedules of drugs; for example, Schedule V drugs are not always monitored (Alliance of States with Prescription Monitoring Programs, 2011). The U.S. Department of Health and Human Services, Health Resources and Services Administration (HRSA) has developed a rolling 12-month client medical profile that can be accessed through the agency that oversees a state's Medicaid program. For example, upon request of the practitioner, the Washington State Department of Social and Health Services will provide a Medicaid patient's list of medications for the last 12 months. A proposed best practice would be to request the list about a week prior to a patient's scheduled visit, then to review it with the patient for medication adherence as well as potential drug abuse issues. While this tactic would not be useful for the transient patient, it may provide useful data for an established patient's care.

Another patient ploy is to be extraordinarily persuasive or dramatic. Patients may create a disturbance in the waiting room hoping to obtain what they want. Patients may expect that the APRN's desire to protect one's professional reputation or decrease the potential discomfort of other clinic patients and staff will cause him/her to acquiesce to their demands (Robbins, 2007).

Many patients are obvious in their quest to obtain medications for inappropriate use while others are more skilled. A patient may appear to be reasonable and initially requests a drug without abuse potential. As the appointments ends, the patient makes an "Oh, by the way" request for a controlled substance used or recommended by a friend or family member. These types of medication requests usually require return visits by the patient for more in-depth assessment. Another approach can be to mispronounce or misspell a drug name in an attempt to feign naïveté (Roscoe, 2004).

Approaches to deal with difficult situations

It is often difficult to have certainty that a patient is abusing a prescription medication. Despite this, healthcare providers maintain the right to decline what they perceive to be an inappropriate medication request (Drug Enforcement Administration, 1999). Viewing the patient with concern-raising behaviors through the lens of a patient with a serious illness may shift the APRN's comfort level in these difficult situations. Suggested approaches to these difficult situations include the following.

- Work with the patient to identify a common goal.
- Where agreement cannot be reached, agree to disagree.
- Reference the chief complaint and help the patient describe how the problem is affecting his or her functioning.
- Use assessment of function to evaluate a patient's progress rather than subjective complaints (McCaffery et al., 2005).
- Assess if the patient is able to awaken easily in the morning.
- Assess if the patient is able to work and meet family obligations.
- Acknowledge the patient and empathize with the struggles.
- Advise the patient about ways he/she can be assisted.
- Avoid becoming defensive as that may escalate patient emotions.
- Even though threats are seldom carried out, involve security or police when one's comfort level is exceeded.

Working with substance abusers

Conversations about drug abuse can be productive if the patient senses the APRN is concerned for his or her interests and speaks nonjudgmentally (Wilford, 1990). Respectfully inquire as to whether the patient believes he or she has an abuse problem with prescription drugs. Maintain a professional demeanor and confront the patient in a gentle, respectful manner. Most patients are likely to respond to an approach that is without judgment or antagonism and avoids maternalistic/paternalistic or infantilizing tones.

If the patient admits that there is a problem, conduct an assessment, discuss readiness for treatment, and when appropriate, refer the patient for treatment. While drug abuse can be difficult to treat, psychological treatments from an increasing number of well-designed randomized controlled trials have demonstrated effectiveness in treating drug dependence (Neavins, Easton, Brotchie, & Carroll, 2008). It is essential that APRNs continue to maintain hope and actively encourage patients with drug abuse issues to seek treatment as they would for all their patients.

A common dilemma is whether to provide some medication to the patient until drug treatment is obtained. Withdrawal from opioids can be debilitating, but is rarely fatal. In contrast, it is essential to carefully guide a patient's withdrawal from benzodiazepines. Depending upon the strength of dosage and length of treatment, it can be extremely difficult to taper patients off benzodiazepines (Childress, 2004). There are currently no Food and Drug Administration (FDA)-approved medications for benzodiazepine withdrawal, but anticonvulsants are frequently used to prevent seizures (Inaba & Cohen, 2007; Kosten & O'Connor, 2003). Resources are available on the Internet for benzodiazepine management and withdrawal (Ashton, 2002).

An evidence-based in-depth resource about withdrawal of benzodiazepines including pharmacokinetics, dependency, and rebound, may be useful to APRNs (Nelson & Chouinard, 1999). The Ashton Manual (2002) is an Internet-based resource for coaching about benzodiazepine management and withdrawal. Because benzodiazepines are a valuable medication in treating a variety of health conditions across specialties, expertise in preventing abuse needs to be balanced with comfort with prescribing these medications appropriately.

When the APRN confronts a patient with a drug abuse problem, it is important to recall that substance abuse is a chronic, relapsing disease. While patients do not always reach recovery with the first attempt at treatment, some eventually succeed. Some may even question whether a provider's earlier refusal of their requests for controlled substances could have hastened treatment (Goldman, 1987).

APRNs have an ethical responsibility to appropriately prescribe, maintain knowledge of controlled substances, and to be alert to patients who may want to manipulate them. In the early 1980s, as part of an effort to more appropriately discipline "misprescribers," the American Medical Association created the Four-D classification: dated, duped, dishonest, and disabled (Longo et al., 2000; Wesson & Smith, 1990). (See Box 5.5.)

To avoid falling into the "dated" category, it is important, particularly if one does not routinely treat conditions that require controlled substances, to maintain prescribing competencies. An APRN is more likely to be "duped" because of gullibility, discom-

> **Box 5.5 AMA four D's of misprescribers**
>
> **Dated**: This refers to prescribers who are out of date regarding knowledge of pharmacology and the differential diagnosis and management of chronic pain, anxiety, insomnia, and addiction.
>
> **Duped**: Most healthcare practitioners are caring, trusting professionals who are trying to help their patients in an open and honest relationship based on mutual respect. Thus, practitioners may be vulnerable to a manipulative patient.
>
> **Disabled**: A disabled prescriber is one with a medical or psychiatric disability, such as chemical dependency or a personality disorder. These prescribers may be less likely to confront patients who are abusing substances out of fear of turning suspicion on themselves. Practitioners also need to be aware of co-dependent traits. Practitioners with co-dependence issues often have difficulty with confronting patients with a similar problem.
>
> **Dishonest**: There are a few prescribers in every geographic area who are willing to write prescriptions for controlled substances in exchange for financial gain. These practitioners should be reported to the appropriate licensing board and other law enforcement agencies.
>
> *Source*: Longo et al., 2000.

fort in confronting patients, or pride that prevents one from seeking appropriate consultation. All practitioners can occasionally be manipulated or "taken in" by a patient's story. The duped provider has a recurring pattern of acquiescing to demands of patients and prescribing drugs in excessive amounts or for longer than necessary.

"Disabled" providers are those whose judgment is impaired by their own illness, alcohol, or drug use. Healthcare practitioners constitute an unusually high-risk group for abuse of controlled substances because of occupational access (Lowinson, Ruiz, & Millman, 2005). The "dishonest" practitioner is one who prescribes willfully for other than medical purposes. Such practitioners are using their license to "deal" drugs rather than for any legitimate purpose and should be barred from the profession (Lowinson et al., 2005). To avoid falling into one of the Four D's, it is critical for the APRN to maintain the essential skill of learning to resist patient pressure to prescribe something when one is not comfortable with the situation.

Diversion and deception

Concern-raising behaviors that may be forms of deception include concealing or pretending to take medications, requesting refills in a shorter period of time than originally prescribed, or claims of lost or stolen medications (Drug Enforcement Administration, 1999; Robbins, 2007). Drug abusers may also use a child or an elderly person to obtain stimulants or pain medications. It is essential for APRNs to be vigilant in assessing whether an adult may be diverting drugs used to treat a child's ADHD or opioid medications prescribed to vulnerable older adults (Robbins, 2007).

It is often difficult to differentiate a patient who might be diverting medications from one who is overusing medications. A urine toxicology screen may be a useful tool to assist with this assessment. Patients who are diverting drugs may claim to take a medication regularly; however, this claim may not be substantiated by urine screening tests.

Drug abusers frequently report lost or stolen medications (Drug Enforcement Administration [DEA], 1999; Wilford, 1990). Patients should be instructed that medications are valuable commodities and should be guarded as carefully as they would guard their wallet. Here is an analogy that emphasizes this point. If a wallet is stolen, no one would expect the bank to refund the money. Likewise, the expectation that lost prescriptions will be resupplied for controlled substances is inappropriate. As with all dimensions of prescribing practice, APRN practitioners need to assess patient safety when making these decisions.

Strategies to prevent diversion

Electronic prescribing has many intentions and benefits, one of which is the reduction of the risk of prescription forgery and alteration (DEA, 2010). However, this new technology is far from universal, and many APRNs have only the written prescription option. A key approach used to address problems with paper prescriptions has become the use of tamper-resistant forms. Increasing attention is focused on avoiding problems that arise from access to blank prescriptions. Security measures include storing prescription forms that are not actively in use in a locked location and limiting the number of prescription forms in use at one time. Some clinicians pre-sign prescriptions for convenience in a busy clinic, a practice that is illegal (Code of the Federal Register, n.d.).

Instructions for a non-pharmacological treatment written on a prescription form may be perceived as more "official" than verbal instructions (e.g., an exercise prescription), thus creating a dilemma for practitioners who utilize this approach. This practice is discouraged because it adds to the risk of forgery (Wilford, 1990).

APRNs can approach challenging situations in a variety of ways. Often there is no "right" way, and it is important that responses are a comfortable fit with a practitioner's interaction style. Comfort, however, develops over time with repeated practice. Because many professionals understandably want to avoid conflict, there is a pervasive need to "learn" appropriate and skillful approaches. The use of specific strategies can provide guidance as APRNs develop expertise in the prevention of diversion. Chapter 4 also includes several additional strategies that can be used for screening.

- Require identification for patients new to the practice.
  - Advise patients this is a standard procedure and obtain a photocopy of the identification.
- Request that patients sign a release of information for their previous practitioners and explain documentation must be received before prescriptions will be provided.
- Assess the patient and develop a diagnosis independent of the prior providers. The assessment should include questions about drug abuse (Longo et al., 2000).
- Ask the patient if he or she has received any prescriptions for controlled substances within the last 30 days and record the patient's response in his or her presence.
- Ask the patient: "How many times in the past year have you used an illegal drug or used a prescription medication for non-medical reasons?"

The above question was 100% sensitive and 73.5% specific (confidence interval = 95%) for the detection of a drug use disorder in a general population of primary care patients (Smith, Schmidt, Allensworth-Davies, & Saitz, 2010).

Documentation is always essential. However, this area of prescribing requires even more careful and extensive documentation of the history, screening questions and responses, examination, and the results of tests to protect one's practice. The decision to prescribe medications should be evidence-based and consider the schedule of the drug, the severity of the symptoms, and potential for drug abuse. If there are concern-raising behaviors, the practitioner can write prescriptions for limited quantities and evaluate the patient frequently until trust is established.

APRNs may be better able to prevent diversion if they are able to identify and avoid common pitfalls. Patients whose goal is to divert drugs can often be threatening and intimidating. These behaviors should not be tolerated by APRNs. Calling a colleague, clinic supervisory staff, or security personnel is essential even if in some occasions the situation never escalates. Practitioners may avoid seeking this support because of the desire to "not bother" someone. In contrast, calling for this type of assistance may communicate to patients one's serious commitment to safety and avoiding manipulation, and serve as a role model for colleagues.

A common mistake, made with the goal to prompt the patient to leave the clinic and end the disruption for other patients and staff, is to acquiesce to the patient's request. Ethical issues along with increased clinician vulnerability may arise when even small amounts of medication are prescribed in the context of intimidation. It is essential to have an established practitioner–patient relationship in order to provide any prescription, but it is especially important with the prescribing of controlled substances. In the absence of such a relationship, it is not appropriate to prescribe scheduled drugs. Many practices authorize only designated prescribers to refill controlled substances.

Legal issues related to prescribing in difficult situations

As APRNs have attained full prescriptive authority, one of the barriers to embracing this authority has been the fear of disciplinary action by regulators (Kaplan & Brown, 2008). Despite this common fear, very little is known about the frequency of action taken against APRNs and most data address physicians only. In one nationwide study of prescription prescribing practices, the conclusion was: "the risk of state medical board disciplinary action against a physician for treating a bona fide patient with opioids for a painful medical condition, in the absence of other misconduct, is virtually nonexistent" (Richard & Reidenberg, 2005, p. 211).

In almost all incidents, disciplinary action against prescribers related to controlled substances instead focused on diversion or practitioner incompetence in areas such as prescribing for an addict without proper assessment (Richard & Reidenberg, 2005). Somewhat related is the example of a malpractice suit brought by a patient who accuses the physician of failing to address behavior obviously reflective of addiction (Steenburgh, 2002).

In Washington State, Schedule II–IV prescriptive authority for APRNs was implemented in 2001. Data regarding APRN disciplinary action between 2001 and 2007 by the Washington State Quality Assurance Commission were reviewed. No action taken against APRNs for overprescribing controlled substances was noted (Kaplan & Brown, 2008). Subsequent to the review, a nurse practitioner was disciplined for care of patients with chronic noncancer pain that fell below the standard of a reasonably competent nurse practitioner placing them at risk of moderate to severe harm. Part of the disciplinary action suspended the provider's Schedule II prescribing privileges for a minimum of 2 years.[1]

A focus on limiting legal risks can increase APRNs' comfort with prescribing. First of all, provide informed consent prior to the prescription of any medication. With controlled substances, the risk of addiction, tolerance, and dependence should be fully disclosed. Additionally, there is a "duty to warn" patients of the risk of driving while taking a medication that can affect alertness (Longo et al., 2000). When needed, it is also useful to consult with an experienced peer or refer to an addiction specialist, a psychopharmacologist, or a pain management specialist.

Patient confidentiality needs to be maintained even when there is a concern with a patient suspected of drug abuse. Consultation may be made with other healthcare professionals regarding a

---

[1] The record for this review is publicly available. Out of respect for privacy, the link to the record is not provided.

patient's visit, treatment, or complaints. However, it is not acceptable to call a provider outside your healthcare organization who does not have an established relationship with the patient to warn about suspected drug abuse (Roscoe, 2004). That may lead to legal action as a violation of the Health Insurance Portability and Accountability Act.

Another strategy for providing clarity in the patient–practitioner relationship is through the use of medication agreements. These are not legal documents and need to have a clear justification. Legal liability may be prevented by clarifying the conditions under which controlled substances will be prescribed (Smith, 2006). Controversy exists around the role, advantages, and limitations associated with medication agreements. Decisions made by a group of practice colleagues can establish consistency about how the group will approach this issue.

Considerable criticism has arisen about providers who use medication agreements with the intent of setting up a plan which would justify the discharge of "problem patients" in their practice. Most practitioners, however, use contracts to clarify conditions of treatment in a way that will benefit both patient and provider. Contracts must be clearly understood in order to use them as a tool, rather than a weapon; it is important to assess the patient's understanding of the consequences of violating the agreement (D'Arcy, 2009). It is also important for the APRN to clearly specify the consequences of violating the agreement. Indicate if a violation will result in the discontinuation of controlled substances or the discontinuation of care. Indicate if there ever are exceptions. Another consideration is whether agreements are required with all patients on controlled substances, patients on long-term therapy with controlled substances, or only those patients who exhibit concern-raising behaviors. The problem with the latter is that some patients do not initially present with concern-raising behaviors at the beginning of treatment. A number of medication agreements exist in the public domain (Department of Social and Health Services, n.d.; Hariharan, Lamb, & Neuner, 2007; Oregon Health and Science University, 2009; Smith, 2006). Alternately, APRNs may choose to create or adapt an agreement.

In summary, patients who present with concern-raising behaviors for substance abuse are a challenge for prescribing practitioners. The astute APRN will be alert to warning signs in patients, be prepared with a strategy for managing the difficult situations these patients create, and act courageously to implement these strategies. All responses are based on a foundation of respect for the patient as well as self-awareness and self-reflection.

MANAGING DIFFICULT PATIENTS WITH SOMATOFORM DISORDERS

Patients who present with physical symptoms or complaints for which there is no organic basis may be experiencing a somatoform disorder. The term *somatoform* covers a group of conditions in the DSM-IV-TR (American Psychiatric Association, 2000) where physical symptoms reported by patients are most likely related to psychological factors unconnected to a specific physical cause. Many APRNs outside those practicing in mental health may not have been exposed to these diagnoses for patients that are likely common across most practice settings. Patients with these conditions require careful management approaches that either mirror or differ from patients who exhibit concern-raising behaviors related to substance abuse.

Diagnosing somatoform disorder

To warrant the diagnosis of somatoform disorder, the symptoms must cause the patient significant impairment or distress. Since patients assume these conditions are caused by medical problems, they typically present in primary care and specialty care rather than in mental health practices. Somatoform disorders are the most common mental disorders presenting in a general practice and are thought to make up 10%–15% of patients (Kroenke, 2009). In one study of a general practice, somatoform disorder was found to make up 16% of the practice. When the criterion of severe clinical impairment was not used, the incidence rose to 22%. Somatoform disorder exceeded the incidence of anxiety disorders at 5.5% and depressive disorders at 4.1% (Waal, Arnold, Eekhof, & Van Hemert, 2004).

The etiological origins of somatoform disorders are unknown. Modern evidence suggests a multifactorial etiology with biological, social, and psychological factors (Mayou, Kirmayer, Simon, Kroenke, & Sharpe, 2005). There is increased evidence that biologic factors are increasingly relevant (Sharpe & Carson, 2001). One hypothesis is that some individuals are more sensitive and therefore amplify visceral and somatic sensations. Both irritable bowel syndrome patients and fibromyalgia patients have been noted to have hypersensitivity to the experimental pain conditions and widespread alteration in central pain processing (Straud, Nagel, Robinson, & Price, 2009; Zhou, Fillingim, Riley, & Verne, 2010).

Amplification of symptoms is also seen during time of psychosocial difficulties and stress. It is generally accepted that social and mental stress not only aggravate physical symptoms but can also trigger physical symptoms in the absence of a physiologic disorder (Barsky, 1992). Occasionally, symptoms are considered to be metaphors, such as chest pain experienced with a "broken heart." Other patients may perceive, usually unconsciously, that symptoms serve a useful purpose (Gillette, 2000). The stigma associated with mental illness may compel patients to seek primary or specialty care for physical symptoms which may be perceived as more socially acceptable. There are also indications that somatoform disorders can run in families, although the nature versus nurture question is not clear. Whatever the etiology, somatoform disorders are frustrating for the clinician and create high levels of dissatisfaction among patients.

It is important to distinguish somatoform disorders from two related disorders, factitious disorder and malingering (American Psychiatric Association, 2000). A factitious disorder is the intentional production or feigning of physical or psychological signs or symptoms. The motivation for the behavior is to assume the sick role. Malingering is the purposeful feigning of physical symptoms for external gain such as economic gain, avoiding legal responsibility, or improving physical well-being. In contrast, with somatoform disorder, there are no obvious gains or incentives for the patient, and the physical symptoms are not willfully adopted or feigned. Somatoform disorders are more likely the result of anxiety and fear (Oyama, Paltoo, & Greengold, 2007).

Managing somatoform disorders

Patients with somatoform disorders may present the APRN with the common dilemma of addressing requests for an unnecessary test or unwarranted medication. A key aspect of management is building a trusting, respectful relationship where a patient experiences the practitioner's caring and compassion. Discussion of the patient's suffering caused by this disorder may be an important part of the conversation. Difficult discussions about including mental health care as part of the treatment plan may then be more successful.

When a patient with somatoform disorder is resistant to mental health therapy, that resistance needs to be carefully explored. Sometimes it may be relatively straightforward to help the patient deal with the anxiety of having to select a psychiatric, mental health APRN from a pool of unfamiliar, perhaps even intimidating healthcare professionals. At other times the resistance may be intractable, and the patient does not desire to come to terms with a health situation.

Several types of therapy for somatoform disorder have been evaluated. Kroenke (2009) performed a meta-analysis of 34 randomized controlled trials focusing on treatment for somatoform disorders. There was strong evidence of the efficacy of cognitive behavioral therapy (CBT) in 11 out of 13 studies; moderate evidence of improvement in three of four studies where psychiatric consultations with written recommendations for the primary care provider (PCP) were provided; and there were promising results for antidepressant medication therapy in three of four studies. Specialized training for the PCP was not effective. Psychotherapeutic interventions other than CBT also merit further study. Several studies show antidepressant therapy is moderately effective (Cloninger & Dokucu, 2008; Sharpe & Carson, 2001). Most of the clinical trials, however, have focused on single treatments. Sometimes, with mental health as well as other chronic conditions, multimodal treatments might be necessary.

Practitioners who understand the potential value of CBT for their patients may need to address resistance to mental health therapy. Resistance is commonly seen among patients with an explanatory model and belief that they have a serious physical problem. Patients may consider psychosocial or psychiatric explanation implausible and misguided (Chamberlain, 2003; Sharpe & Carson, 2001). Given the lack of clarity in the etiology of somatoform disorders and suggestion of possible biological origins, these patients may be correct. Healthcare providers often feel frustrated

---

Box 5.6 Practice management strategies for somatoform disorders

- Recognize that patients may have physical symptoms for which there is no medical explanation, without malingering or feigning symptoms.
- Schedule regular, brief follow-up office visits with the patient.
  - Conduct a brief physical examination to provide comfort and reassurance.
  - Avoid unnecessary tests, surgeries, and referrals.
  - Prescribe medications with caution and for specific indications.
- Limit frequent telephone calls and "urgent" visits. Advise the patient to keep a list of concerns to discuss at the next regularly scheduled visit.
- Focus interventions on functioning and management of the disorder, not on diagnosis and cure. Issues to be addressed may include:
  - Stress reduction
  - Lifestyle modification.
- Include the patient's family in the development of the treatment plan if appropriate and possible.
- Treat comorbid physical and psychiatric disorders with appropriate interventions.

---

or guilty when patients do not recover or improve. A supportive approach can provide comfort to the patient and satisfaction for the provider (Gillette, 2000).

Patients with somatoform disorder may benefit from a structured approach to interactions with their primary and specialty care providers (see Box 5.6). Scheduled appointments demonstrate to the patient that the APRN takes his or her concerns seriously. At the same time, avoiding appointments on demand may reduce the possibility of reinforcing the "sick" role among patients with somatoform disorder.

Regardless of the patient's openness to appropriate treatment, APRNs must set boundaries and discuss the rationale for limiting unnecessary diagnostic tests or medications and how the patient's quality of care could be affected. It is important for APRNs to develop comfort and skill with requests for unnecessary care and learn to avoid the associated pitfalls which include exposure of the patient to potential health risks, utilization of financial resources, and increased demands on the healthcare system.

RESPONDING TO A REQUEST FOR AN INAPPROPRIATE TREATMENT

As discussed in detail in Chapter 6, direct-to-consumer advertising coupled with extensive health information on the Internet and media coverage of health care has changed the nature of interactions between APRNs and patients. This information, whether or not it is accurate, has prompted many patients to request a medication, diagnostic test, or treatment they have read about or seen in the media. Sometimes, these requests are appropriate, and other times they are not. Patients make inappropriate requests for a variety of reasons and motivations. Many patients legitimately believe these requests are in their best interest and do not understand why the APRN does not agree. APRNs, in contrast, do not want to seem cold, uncaring, or withholding of appropriate treatments. There is little in the literature to guide APRNs on how to "just say no."

An example of one approach to a difficult situation could be to discuss with the patient how acquiescence to the request could be viewed as malpractice by colleagues or health systems. Similarly, it may be useful to help the patient understand the new imperatives of the current healthcare arena such as evidence-based practice, clinical guidelines, professional organization recommendation and institutional policy that guides or limits practitioners. Reinforcing the message that appropriate care is quality care and can lead to greater patient satisfaction is a particularly relevant foundation for prescribing medications (see Box 5.7). Speaking succinctly with authority with an evidence-based rationale is often met with a positive response. Patients may also respond well when they are convinced that the APRN has put the patient's interests first.

Online resources and printed materials can also be useful to review with patients. For example, a very common request in outpatient clinics and office practice settings is for antibiotics to treat a viral respiratory infection. Education about the nature of viral illnesses often manages these requests. The Centers for Disease Control and Prevention (CDC) has developed resource materials

---

Box 5.7 Strategies to say no

Keep it simple: Provide a concise medical explanation at a level the patient can understand. Repeat if necessary, but do not provide extensive or defensive explanations.

Accept responsibility for the decision: This is your decision so do not disempower yourself by blaming an employer, the Drug Enforcement Administration, or some other authority. While it is appropriate to cite standards of practice, here again, a lengthy explanation is not warranted.

Understand why you are making the decision: If you do not have good rationale for the clinical decision you are making, it will be difficult to make it clear to the patient. However, there are those times when an expert APRN will be guided by experience and intuition. In these instances, it might be appropriate to buy time. Tell the patient you want to think about the request or seek consultation from a trusted colleague. Patients by and large appreciate that you do not want to do anything that might cause them harm.

Put the patient first: Telling patients there is an important reason not to prescribe or provide a treatment is generally effective.

Agree to disagree: There are times when a patient is willing to "take the risk" and is insistent upon their preferred mode of treatment. When an APRN reaches an impasse with a patient, it can be interpreted as a genuine disagreement. Suggest that you agree to disagree and underscore your respect for them and their point of view. However, let them know that you also have respect for yourself and will not do what you believe to be harmful to them or in your estimation is poor nursing practice.

---

for clinicians and patients that can be accessed on the CDC website (Centers for Disease Control and Prevention, 2011). Their campaign called "Get Smart: Know When Antibiotics Work" was developed to help providers deal with the problem of antibiotic resistance. Increasingly, as evidence-based practice and research about the translation of evidence to practice take hold, there is a deepening awareness that saying no to patients often involves a difficult clinical conversation. Patient requests may cause an anxiety-provoking situation for some APRNs. However, polite, firm, direct, and brief explanations with a clear decision generally provide greater satisfaction to both parties. Many practitioners were educated prior to this new evidence-oriented environment; many in a time when patients and practitioners worked with the understanding that "the provider knows best." A new set of negotiation, collaboration, and conflict resolution skills is now an essential part of the APRN toolkit to manage the complex arena of prescribing medications.

THE DECISION TO NOT ACCEPT TREATMENT RECOMMENDATIONS

The decision not to accept healthcare provider recommendations regarding treatment by patients is more the norm than the exception. Sackett was one of the first to study patients' decisions to take medications. He found that patients take medications as prescribed an estimated 50%–60% of the time (Sackett & Snow, 1979). Vermeire, Hearnshaw, Van Royen, and Denekens (2001) conducted a review of research about treatment adherence by patients. There are serious problems with methods for generating valid and reliable data to give accurate estimates of patient adherence. However, they did estimate that "noncompliance" can be expected with 30%–50% of all patients regardless of the disease, prognosis, or setting (Vermeire et al., 2001). In addition to problematic follow through about medications, resistance to recommendations in regard to diet, exercise, and cessation of the use of tobacco products and other harmful substances commonly occurs.

It can be very difficult for a patient to do a risk–benefit analysis about a medication they have never taken. They may have little sense of the "future benefit" or how they may feel if a medication was effective. Without the ability to imagine feeling better, current decision making can be clouded by anxiety about side effects or fear of the unknown. Some patients may have spiritual, religious, cultural, or family value systems that emphasize acceptance of all life circumstances that occur. Other patients approach their lives with an overall passivity or a hypersensitization to using medication from a family history of medication abuse. Being proactive about improving one's future health through medication therapy can be unacceptable or unimaginable to some patients. The APRN's core philosophy of patient-centered care can help prevent these situations from becoming "difficult patient situations."

The choice triad

Resistance to requests and recommendations occurs either when the patient does not do what the practitioner advises or the provider does not do what the patient desires. In his book, *Improving Medication Adherence*, Shea (2006) outlines what he refers to as the "Choice Triad" which was created by nurses and doctors to identify when they themselves would take medications.

1. They feel there is something wrong with them.
2. They feel motivated to try to get help with what is wrong (or to prevent future problems from arising) through the use of medication.
3. They believe that the benefits of taking the medication will, in the long run, outweigh the risks.

Shea discusses the language used to describe when patients decide not to take medication or follow treatment recommendations. Use of the term *noncompliance* implies the APRN is the decision maker and has authority while the patient is obligated to act. Nonadherence is another commonly used term; however, it still does not address the collaborative nature of the therapeutic relationship. Shea proposes using the term *medication interest* as the core concept in discussions with patients. He suggests an approach to the patient that embraces collaboration, for example: "Together we want to find a medicine that you are genuinely interested in taking because it makes you feel better" (p. 38).

Shea suggests the *Choice Triad* as a framework for discussing medications with patients. It is important to first assess if the patient feels something is wrong. For example, a patient with schizophrenia who experiences anosognosia will likely not take a medication voluntarily. Many hypertensive patients do not experience symptoms, do not understand or believe the possible consequences, or do not know someone with untreated hypertension who has had a stroke or heart attack. They may not view elevated blood pressure as a health threat. The patient who does not believe something is wrong will not want to take an antipsychotic that might induce tardive dyskinesia or metabolic syndrome. From the patient's point of view, these preferences are understandable.

Box 5.8 Case example: patient-centered care

A family nurse practitioner (FNP) was exploring the goals and ambitions held by a 36-year-old man with type 2 diabetes and hypertension. The FNP discovered that while she was focused on lowering the patient's blood glucose and blood pressure, the patient was not focused on this topic. Instead, his focus in life was getting a promotion at work, preparing for fatherhood, and purchasing a new home. This led to a productive discussion of ways to achieve his goals, none of which directly related to taking medications. However, he was able to identify how managing his medications better might assist him in working toward his goals.

The second tenet of the *Choice Triad* guides the APRN to identify what the patient wants (see Box 5.8). In addition to focusing on the patient's hopes and dreams, it is also helpful to discuss what is most discouraging. For example, the joy in relief from depression or hypertension may be dampened if the patient develops sexual dysfunction. They may value a satisfying sexual life as more important than treating elevated blood pressure, anxiety, or depression.

The third tenet of the *Choice Triad* relates to what patients may have to give up or experience to treat their disease. Patients are often willing to endure some discomfort such as mild, transient side effects from a medication if the situation will improve. If not forewarned, the patient may assume the medication is making him worse and not better. In one study, patients who received specific educational messages were also more likely to accept a prescribed medication regimen (Lin et al., 1995). Another study found the communication style of the provider and client satisfaction were both predictive of higher medication interest (Bultman & Svarstad, 2000). In an article dealing with difficult patients, Miksanek (2008) emphasized communication and hope.

> To continue being blunt, it's all about how . . . [providers] and patients related to one another. And the problem with a difficult patient isn't just the patient. It's also [the provider]. Difficult patients and their [providers] fail each other. We flop together. We lose hope. There is no more

worthless [provider] than one who has lost all hope. Same holds true for a patient. (p. 1428)

Patient-centered care can help providers and patients remain hopeful and connected to each other. If patients believe they need help, if they are consulted about the nature of the problem, and if they are included in the discussion of the risks and benefits, they are more likely to actively participate and engage in treatment recommendations. Placing the patient at the center of the treatment plan creates a working alliance between the APRN and patient that limits the frustrations of both.

CONCLUSION

The important theme throughout this chapter is that there are "difficult situations" rather than "difficult patients." Often, these are not patient problems but rather situations where the APRN lacks knowledge or skills to manage the situation. Through self-awareness, ethical treatment, and increased skill building, APRNs can learn to manage many of the common communication problems in the patient–nurse relationship.

Communication problems in health care may arise as providers focus on diseases and their management, rather than on people, their lives, and their health problems (Lewin, Skea, Entwistle, Zwarenstein, & Dick, 2001). These concepts of holistic care are the quintessential hallmark of nursing and often are described as part of nursing's unique perspective about the value of prescriber–patient partnerships. As with all prescribers, APRN–patient interactions surrounding medication and prescribing are inherently vulnerable to all the challenges previously discussed. Even with the increasing pace of practice today, APRNs can prioritize their communication with patients, especially surrounding prescribing, as a priority that cannot be compromised. Rewards are often evident in the APRN's experience of establishing strong connections with people and in the deep satisfaction of making a difference.

REFERENCES

Alliance of States with Prescription Monitoring Programs. (2011). Retrieved from http://www.pmpalliance.org/

Amanatullah, E. T., & Morris, M. W. (2010). Negotiating gender roles: Gender differences in assertive negotiating are mediated by women's fear of backlash and attenuated when negotiating on behalf of others. *Journal of Personality and Social Psychology, 98*(2), 256–267.

American Nurses Association. (2001). Code of ethics for nurses with interpretive statements. Retrieved from http://www.ananursingethics.org/nursingethics.htm#prov1

American Psychiatric Association. (2000). *Diagnostic and statistical manual of mental disorders* (4th ed.). Washington DC: Author.

American Society for Pain Management Nursing [ASPMN]. (2011). *Position statement: Pain management in patients with substance abuse and addictive disease.* Lenexa, KS: Author. May be Retrieved from http://www.aspmn.org

Anderson, D. L., Hoop, J. G., & Roberts, L. W. (2009). The psychiatric interview. In L. Roberts, J. Hoop, & T. Heinrich (Eds.), *Clinical psychiatry essentials* (pp. 23–37). Philadelphia: Wolters Kluver/Lippincott, Williams & Wilkins.

Ashton, C. H. (2002). Benzodiazepines: How they work and how to withdraw. Retrieved from http://www.benzo.org.uk/manual/

Barsky, A. J. (1992). Amplification, somatization, and the somatoform disorders. *Psychosomatics, 33*(1), 28–34.

Benner, P., & Tanner, C. (1987). Clinical judgment: How expert nurses use intuition. *American Journal of Nursing, 87*(1), 23–34.

Brown, M. A., & Draye, M. A. (2003). The experiences of pioneer nurse practitioners in establishing advanced practice roles. *Journal of Nursing Scholarship, 35*(4), 389–395.

Bultman, D., & Svarstad, B. (2000). Effects of physician communication style on client medication beliefs and adherence with antidepressant treatment. *Patient Education and Counseling, 40*(2), 173–185.

Centers for Disease Control and Prevention. (2011). Get smart: Know when antibiotics work. Retrieved from http://www.cdc.gov/getsmart/

Chamberlain, J. R. (2003). Approaches to somatoform disorders in primary care. *Somatoform Disorders, 3*(8), 438–447.

Childress, K. (2004). Drug seeking patients: How to spot them, treat them, and protect your practice. *Physicians Practice, 14*(9).

Retrieved from http://www.physicianspractice.com/display/article/1462168/1588715

Cloninger, C. R., & Dokucu, M. (2008). Somatoform and dissociative disorders. In S. Fatemi, & P. Clayton (Eds.), *The medical basis of psychiatry* (pp. 181–194). New Jersey: Humana Press.

Code of the Federal Register. (n.d.). §1306.05 Manner of issuance of prescriptions. Retrieved from http://edocket.access.gpo.gov/cfr_2010/aprqtr/pdf/21cfr1306.05.pdf

D'Arcy, Y. (2009). Be in the know about pain management. *The Nurse Practitioner, 34*(4), 43–47.

Department of Social and Health Services. (n.d.). Helping patients with drug use disorders. Retrieved from http://www.dshs.wa.gov/pdf/dbhr/CD%20ScreeningGuideforMedicalProf.pdf

Driscoll, J., & Teh, B. (2001). The potential of reflective practice to develop individual orthopaedic nurse practitioners and their practice. *Journal of Orthopaedic Nursing, 5*(2), 95–103.

Drug Enforcement Administration. (1999). Don't be scammed by a drug abuser. Retrieved from http://www.deadiversion.usdoj.gov/pubs/brochures/drugabuser.htm

Drug Enforcement Administration. (2010). Economic impact analysis of the interim final electronic prescription rule. Retrieved from http://www.deadiversion.usdoj.gov/ecomm/e_rx/eia_dea_218.pdf

Duffy, A. (2007). A concept analysis of reflective practice: Determining its value to nurses. *British Journal of Nursing, 16*(22), 1400–1407.

Fisher, F. B. (2004). Interpretation of "aberrant" drug-related behaviors. *Journal of American Physicians and Surgeons, 9*(1), 25–28.

Fowler, M. (2000). A new code of ethics for nurses. *American Journal of Nursing, 100*(7), 69–72.

Gillette, R. D. (2000). "Problem patients": A fresh look at an old vexation. *American Academy of Family Physicians.* Retrieved from http://www.aafp.org/fpm/20000700/57prob.html

Goldman, B. (1987). Confronting the prescription drug addict: Doctors must learn to say no. *Canadian Medical Association Journal, 136*(5), 871–876.

Haas, L. J., Leiser, J. P., Magill, M. K., & Sanyer, O. N. (2005). Management of the difficult patient. *American Family Physician, 72*(10), 2063–2068.

Hariharan, J., Lamb, G. C., & Neuner, J. M. (2007). Long-term opioid contract use for chronic pain management in primary care practice: A five year experience. *Journal of General Internal Medicine*, *22*(4), 485–490.

Inaba, D. S., & Cohen, W. E. (2007). *Uppers, downers, all arounders* (6th ed.). Medford, OR: CNS Productions.

Jones, A. C. (2004). Transference and countertransference. *Perspectives in Psychiatric Care*, *40*(1), 13–19.

Jones, J. M. (2010). Nurses top honesty and ethics list for 11th year. Retrieved from http://www.gallup.com/poll/145043/Nurses-Top-Honesty-Ethics-List-11-Year.aspx

Kaplan, L., & Brown, M. A. (2008). Prescribing controlled substances: Perceptions, realities, and experiences in Washington state. *The American Journal for Nurse Practitioners*, *12*(3), 44–53.

Keaveney, R. (2004). Dealing with problem patients. *Physicians Practice*, *14*(3). Retrieved from http://www.physicianspractice.com

Koekkoek, B., van Meijel, B., & Hutschemaekers, G. (2006). "Difficult patients" in mental health care: A review. *Psychiatric Services*, *57*(6), 795–802.

Kosten, T. R., & O'Connor, P. G. (2003). Current concepts: Management of drug and alcohol withdrawal. *New England Journal of Medicine*, *348*(18), 1786–1795, 1831–1832.

Kroenke, K. (2009). Efficacy of treatment for somatoform disorders: A review of randomized controlled trials. *The Journal of Lifelong Learning in Psychiatry*, *7*(3), 414–423.

Lewin, S., Skea, Z., Entwistle, V., Zwarenstein, M., & Dick, J. (2001). Interventions for providers to promote a patient-centered approach in clinical consultations. *Cochrane Database Of Systematic Reviews*, (4). Retrieved from EBSCO*host*.

Lin, E. H., von Korff, M., Katon, W., Bush, T., Simon, G. E., Walker, E., & Robinson, P. (1995). The role of the primary care physician in patients' adherence to antidepressant therapy. *Medical Care*, *33*(1), 67–74.

Longo, L. P., Parran, T., Jr., Johnson, B., & Kinsey, W. (2000). Addiction: Part II. Identification and management of the drug-seeking patient. *American Family Physician*, *61*(8), 2401–2409. Retrieved from http://www.aafp.org/afp/20000415/2401.html

Lowinson, J. H., Ruiz, P., & Millman, R. B. (2005). *Substance abuse: A comprehensive textbook*. Philadelphia: Lippincott, Williams, & Wilkins.

Mayou, R., Kirmayer, L. J., Simon, G., Kroenke, K., & Sharpe, M. (2005). Somatoform disorders: Time for a new approach in DSM-V. *American Journal of Psychiatry, 162*(5), 847–855.

McCaffery, M., Grimm, M. A., Pasero, C., Ferrell, B., & Uman, G. (2005). On the meaning of "drug seeking." *Pain Management Nursing, 6*(4), 122–136.

Miksanek, T. (2008). On caring for "difficult" patients. *Health Affairs, 27*(5), 1422–1428.

National Institute on Drug Abuse. Preventing and recognizing prescription drug abuse. Retrieved from http://www.nida.nih.gov/ResearchReports/Prescription/prescription6.html

Neavins, T. M., Easton, C. J., Brotchie, J., & Carroll, K. M. (2008). Empirically validated psychologic therapies for drug dependence. In P. Tyrer, & K. Silk (Eds.), *Cambridge textbook of effective treatments in psychiatry* (pp. 353–368). New York: Cambridge University Press.

Nelson, J., & Chouinard, G. (1999). Guidelines for clinical use of benzodiazepines: Pharmacokinetics, dependency, rebound, and withdrawal. *Canadian Journal of Pharmacology, 6*(2), 69–83.

O'Kelly, G. (1998). Countertransference in the nurse-patient relationship: A review of the literature. *Journal of Advanced Nursing, 28*(2), 391–397.

O'Malley, P. O. (2010). Prescription and over-the-counter drug and substance abuse: Something available for every age, anytime and anywhere. *Clinical Nurse Specialist, 24*(6), 286–288.

Oregon Health and Science University. (2009). Principles of prescribing opioids. Retrieved from http://www.ohsu.edu/xd/about/news_events/news/2009/opioidpaindrugguidelines.cfm?WT_rank=

Oyama, O., Paltoo, C., & Greengold, J. (2007). Somatoform disorders. *American Family Physician., 76*(9), 1333–1338.

Patient. (2011). In Merriam-Webster dictionary. Retrieved from http://mw1.merriam-webster.com/dictionary/patient

Pearson, L. (2001). The clinician-patient experience: Understanding transference and countertransference. *The Nurse Practitioner, 26*(6), 8–9.

Peplau, H. (1951). *Interpersonal relations in nursing*. New York: G.P. Putman's Sons.

Richard, J., & Reidenberg, M. M. (2005). The risk of disciplinary action by state medical boards. *Journal of Pain and Symptom Management, 29*(2), 206–212.

Robbins, A. M. P. (2007). How to spot drug seekers in the emergency room setting. Retrieved from http://www.associated content.com/article/286750/how_to_spot_drug_seekers_in_the_emergency.html?cat=71

Roberts, L. W., & Dyer, A. R. (2003). Caring for "difficult" patients. *Focus, 1*(4), 453–458.

Roscoe, M. S. (2004). The drug-seeking patient. *Clinician Reviews, 14*(2), 51–58. Retrieved from http://www.clinicianreviews.com/index.asp?page=8_198.xml

Sackett, D. L., & Snow, J. C. (1979). The magnitude of adherence and nonadherence. In R. Haynes, D. Sackett, & D. Taylor (Eds.), *Adherence in health care* (pp. 11–22). Baltimore, MD: Johns Hopkins University Press.

Sharpe, M., & Carson, A. (2001). "Unexplained" somatic symptoms, functional syndromes, and somatization: Do we need a paradigm shift? *Annals of Internal Medicine, 134*(9), 926–930.

Shea, S. C. (2006). *Improving medication adherence*. Philadelphia: Lippincott Williams & Wilkins.

Smith, P. (2006). Feature: Pain patients, pain contracts, and the war on drugs. 457: 10/12/2006. Retrieved from http://stop thedrugwar.org/chronicle/2006/oct/12/feature_painpatients_pain_contr

Smith, P., Schmidt, S., Allensworth-Davies, D., & Saitz, R. (2010). A single-question screening test for drug use in primary care. *Archives of Internal Medicine, 170*(13), 1155–1160.

van Steenburgh, J. (2002). Tips to spot patients who abuse prescriptions drugs. *ACP-ASIM Observer*. Retrieved from http://www.acpinternist.org/archives/2002/04/drug_abuse.htm

Straud, R., Nagel, S., Robinson, M. E., & Price, D. D. (2009). Enhanced central pain processing of fibromyalgia patients is maintained by muscle afferent input: A randomized, double-blind, placebo-controlled study. *Pain, 145*(1–2), 96–104.

Stuart, G. W. (2009). *Principles and practice of psychiatric nursing*. St. Louis, MO: Mosby Elsevier.

Substance Abuse and Mental Health Services Administration [SAMHSA]. (2008). Types of illicit drug use. Retrieved from http://www.oas.samhsa.gov/NSDUH/2k8NSDUH/tabs/Sect1seTabs1to46.htm#Tab1.1C

Vermeire, E., Hearnshaw, H., Van Royen, P., & Denekens, J. (2001). Patient adherence to treatment: Three decades of research. A comprehensive review. *Journal of Clinical Pharmacy and Therapeutics, 26,* 331–342.

de Waal, M. W. M., Arnold, I. A., Eekhof, J. A. H., & Van Hemert, A. M. (2004). Somatoform disorders in general practice: Prevalence, functional impairment and comorbidity with anxiety and depressive disorders. *The British Journal of Psychiatry, 184*(6), 470–476.

Wesson, D. R., & Smith, D. E. (1990). Prescription drug-abuse patient, physician, and cultural responsibilities. *Western Journal of Medicine, 152*(5), 613–616.

Wilford, B. B. (1990). Abuse of prescription drugs. *The Western Journal of Medicine, 152*(5), 609–612.

Zhou, Q., Fillingim, R. B., Riley, J. L., & Verne, G. N. (2010). Ischemic hypersensitivity in irritable bowel syndrome patients. *Pain Medicine, 11*(11), 1619–1627.

The Influences of Pharmaceutical Marketing on APRN Prescribing

6

Elissa Ladd

> This chapter provides a comprehensive discussion of the characteristics of pharmaceutical marketing and will highlight the impact that marketing can have on the prescribing behaviors of healthcare professionals. Both direct and indirect activities of pharmaceutical marketing are described.

If I learned that my doctor was getting his(her) information from industry-paid lecturers, in seminars sponsored by drug companies, or from reprints selectively given to him(her) from drug reps, I'd get another doctor.

Dr. Jerome Kassirer, Former Editor, *New England Journal of Medicine*
(personal communication, June 2010)

HISTORICAL CONTEXT

The marketing of pharmaceutical agents has become increasingly controversial and is the topic of extensive debate in the health care, social science, and policy literature. However, this controversy must be considered first within the overall context of the history of drug marketing in the United States. Current drug advertising is generally directed to prescribing professionals such as physicians, advanced practice registered nurses (APRNs), and physician

The Advanced Practice Registered Nurse as a Prescriber, First Edition. Marie Annette Brown, Louise Kaplan.
© 2012 John Wiley & Sons, Ltd. Published 2012 by John Wiley & Sons, Ltd.

assistants (PAs). This marketing approach was born of the post World War II renaissance of drug development and approval. With a flood of new medications entering the market, pharmaceutical companies accelerated marketing to sell these products (Podalsky & Green, 2008).

Pharmaceutical marketing has become ubiquitous in today's society. From detailing by representatives in offices and professional meetings to advertisements in print and televised media, professionals and consumers alike receive a substantial amount of information about pharmaceutical agents from industry sources.

DIRECT MARKETING ACTIVITIES

Over the past 20 years, pharmaceutical companies have marketed medications in a variety of ways. These include advertising directly to prescribers in professional journals, face-to-face office-based detailing by pharmaceutical sales representatives, distribution of samples, paid lectures at professional meetings, and electronic or postal promotions (Gagnon & Lexchin, 2008; Suffrin & Ross, 2008).

Direct to prescriber marketing

Most industries that sell products market their goods and/or services directly to the consumer who is making the purchasing decision. The dynamics of marketing in the pharmaceutical industry, however, are different. While the decision to purchase the medication is made by the patient, the decision regarding which product to chose is made by the prescriber. As a consequence, the predominant focus of pharmaceutical marketing is aimed at the health professional who has the legal authority to prescribe pharmaceutical products.

Detailing

The practice of pharmaceutical detailing has been a predominant sales strategy utilized by the industry since the early 1950s. At that time, pharmaceutical companies established a robust pipeline of brand-name prescription-only pharmaceuticals. As a result, more efficient marketing strategies were developed to influence prescribing patterns (Greene, 2007). Placement of drug advertisements in key medical journals proved to be an efficient method for delivering information on their products. Drug companies soon realized that pharmaceutical "salesmen," who later would be renamed "representatives," were effective messengers for product data and materials.

This cadre of scrupulously groomed sales representatives became the face of the industry. Their presentation and etiquette was expected to be "suitable" for physician's offices and hospitals. Great attention was paid to scripted presentations and emphasis on the "educational" as opposed to the "sales" nature of the calls (Greene, 2004). The activities of these early drug sales representatives quickly evolved into what was considered a "professional service" that fulfilled vital educational functions in the medical profession, from the dissemination of information on new products to the overt presence in medical schools and residency programs. However, the ultimate goal of detailing to prescribers has consistently been sales as opposed to education.

The effectiveness of pharmaceutical detailing was evidenced by the rapid proliferation of pharmaceutical sales representatives over the last two decades. At its peak in 2007, the number of industry sales representatives in the United States was estimated to be approximately 102,000 (O'Reilly, 2009). The money spent by the pharmaceutical industry for detailing alone in 2004 was estimated to be between \$7.3 and \$24.4 billion (Gagnon & Lexchin, 2008). Up until 2007, the pharmaceutical industry relied heavily on the distribution by detailers of free gifts such as pens, pads, sticky notes, clocks, and ubiquitous meals. These provided an effective strategy to develop and augment relationships with prescribers. However, because of growing concern about the ethical implications of this gifting strategy to prescribers, this practice has been significantly curtailed by both voluntary and statutory guidelines.

In 2008, the Pharmaceutical Research and Manufacturers of America (PhRMA) updated voluntary guidelines that regulated its relationship with healthcare providers. This ended the practice of small gift giving (pens, pads, clocks, etc.) that was deemed to be "noneducational," as well as the provision of restaurant meals to healthcare providers (Pharmaceutical Research and Manufacturers of American [PhRMA], 2008). The PhRMA code, however, continues to allow meals that are provided in conjunction with informational sessions in medical offices and other practice settings. Box 6.1 contains several sections of the code which can be reviewed in

---

Box 6.1 Selected sections of the code on interactions with healthcare professionals

1. Basis of Interactions

Our relationships with healthcare professionals are regulated by multiple entities and are intended to benefit patients and to enhance the practice of medicine. Interactions should be focused on informing healthcare professionals about products, providing scientific and educational information, and supporting medical education.

Promotional materials provided to healthcare professionals by or on behalf of a company should: (1) be accurate and not misleading; (2) make claims about a product only when properly substantiated; (3) reflect the balance between risks and benefits; and (4) be consistent with all other Food and Drug Administration (FDA) requirements governing such communications.

2. Informational Presentations by Pharmaceutical Company Representatives and Accompanying Meals

Informational presentations and discussions by industry representatives and others speaking on behalf of a company provide healthcare providers with valuable scientific and clinical information about medicines that may lead to improved patient care. In order to provide important scientific information and to respect healthcare professionals' abilities to manage their schedules and provide patient care, company representatives may take the opportunity to present information during healthcare professionals' working day, including mealtimes.

In connection with such presentations or discussions, it is appropriate for occasional meals to be offered as a business courtesy to the healthcare professionals as well as members of their staff attending presentations, so long as the presentations provide scientific or educational value and the meals (1) are modest as judged by local standards; (2) are not part of an entertainment or recreational event; and (3) are provided in a manner conducive to informational communication.

Any such meals offered in connection with informational presentations made by field sales representatives or their immediate managers should also be limited to in-office or in-hospital settings.

Inclusion of a healthcare professional's spouse or other guest in a meal accompanying an informational presentation made by or on behalf of a company is not appropriate. Offering "take-out" meals or meals to be eaten without a company representative being present (such as "dine and dash" programs) is not appropriate.

3. Prohibition on Entertainment and Recreation

Company interactions with healthcare professionals are professional in nature and are intended to facilitate the exchange of medical or scientific information that will benefit patient care. To ensure the appropriate focus on education and informational exchange and to avoid the appearance of impropriety, companies should not provide any entertainment or recreational items, such as tickets to the theater or sporting events, sporting equipment, or leisure or vacation trips, to any healthcare professional who is not a salaried employee of the company. Such entertainment or recreational benefits should not be offered, regardless of (1) the value of the items; (2) whether the company engages the healthcare professional as a speaker or consultant; or (3) whether the entertainment or recreation is secondary to an educational purpose.

Modest, occasional meals are permitted as long as they are offered in the appropriate circumstances and venues as described in relevant sections of this Code.

4. Pharmaceutical Company Support for Continuing Medical Education (CME)

CME, also known as independent medical education (IME), helps physicians and other medical professionals to obtain information and insights that can contribute to the improvement of patient care, and therefore, financial support from companies is appropriate. Such financial support for CME is intended to support education on a full range of treatment options and not to promote a particular medicine. Accordingly, a company should separate its CME grant-making functions from its sales and marketing departments. In addition, a company should develop objective criteria for making CME grant decisions to ensure that the program funded by the company is a bona fide educational program and that the financial support is not an inducement to prescribe or recommend a particular medicine or course of treatment.

Since the giving of any subsidy directly to a healthcare professional by a company may be viewed as an inappropriate cash gift, any financial support should be given to the CME provider, which, in turn, can use the money to reduce the overall CME registration fee for all participants. The company should respect the independent judgment of the CME provider and should follow standards for commercial support established by the Accreditation Council for Continuing Medical Education (ACCME) or other entity that may accredit the CME. When companies underwrite CME, responsibility for and control over the selection of content, faculty, educational methods, materials, and venue

Continued

belongs to the organizers of the conferences or meetings in accordance with their guidelines. The company should not provide any advice or guidance to the CME provider, even if asked by the provider, regarding the content or faculty for a particular CME program funded by the company.

Financial support should not be offered for the costs of travel, lodging, or other personal expenses of nonfaculty healthcare professionals attending CME, either directly to the individuals participating in the event or indirectly to the event's sponsor (except as set out in Section 9 below). Similarly, funding should not be offered to compensate for the time spent by healthcare professionals participating in the CME event.

A company should not provide meals directly at CME events, except that a CME provider at its own discretion may apply the financial support provided by a company for a CME event to provide meals for all participants.

Source: Reprinted from sections of the Code on Interactions with Healthcare Professionals (2009), with permission from the Pharmaceutical Research and Manufacturers of America. For the most up-to-date information, visit www.phrma.org.

its entirety at: http://www.phrma.org/sites/default/files/108/phrma_marketing_code_2008.pdf.

In addition, several states have enacted their own statutes. In 2009, Massachusetts implemented one of the strictest laws in the country in regard to the interface between the pharmaceutical industry and the healthcare professionals. It is significant that the law specifies physician, dentist, and nurse practitioner prescribers. Among other activities, the law prohibits meals that (1) do not include an informational presentation; (2) are offered outside a healthcare professional's office; and (3) are provided to the spouse or guest of a healthcare professional (Zick, 2009). Other states and jurisdictions, including Minnesota, Vermont, and the District of Columbia have enacted similar statutes, and it is presumed that this trend will continue.

Samples

The use of samples by prescribers has been a long-standing practice in many healthcare offices and clinics. The merit of dispensing free sample medications to patients involves two primary rationales. First, it enables the patient to "try out" a new cutting-edge pharmaceutical without committing to a full prescription. Second, samples may also allow patients with limited resources and/or lack of insurance to access expensive medications they are unable to afford. Samples are sometimes considered to be a "pharmaceutical safety net." Many prescribers believe that "the practice of providing free drug samples is based on the tacit assumption that 'sampling' does more good than harm" (Chimonas & Kassirer, 2009, p. 1).

These justifications, however, frequently overshadow the fact that samples are not distributed by pharmaceutical companies as charitable gestures, but instead are used as a very effective marketing tool for new expensive patented drugs. The cost of samples, in fact, is a part of marketing budgets and is not a charitable donation made by the company. These costs are considerable. The retail cost of drug samples went from $4.9 billion in 1996 to $16.4 billion in 2004 (Donahue, Cevaso, & Rosenthal, 2007; Rosenthal, Berndt, Donahue, Frank, & Epstein, 2002).

The use of free drug samples by prescribers has become increasingly controversial. Numerous studies suggest that samples affect the prescribing behaviors of physicians, and there are few studies of other health professionals. The immediate access to samples influences physicians to prescribe drugs other than their preferred choice (Chew et al., 2000); to prescribe more expensive name brand drugs (Adair & Holmgren, 2005); and to prescribe drugs that differed from evidence-based guidelines (Boltri, Gordon, & Vogel, 2002). Moreover, samples have been found to have a negative impact on the provision of quality care (Chimonas & Kassirer, 2009).

Drug samples dispensed by providers rarely are accompanied by instructions on drug administration, side effects, and potential drug interactions that a patient would normally receive from a pharmacist. Also, samples are often newly marketed products whose side effects may not yet be identified. Vioxx, for example, was the most widely distributed sample drug three years after its introduction. Subsequently, it was withdrawn from the market when it became associated with an excess risk of myocardial infarction and stroke (Topol, 2004). This demonstrates the possibility that the safety profile of newer, highly sampled drugs may not be completely apparent during the period shortly after release.

Drug samples have been found to contribute to escalating healthcare costs. Prescription drug spending rose more than five-fold between the years 1990 and 2006, and totaled over $200 billion. It is expected to reach over $515 billion by the year 2017, an increase of 138% (Kaiser Family Foundation, 2008a). A recent estimate of the cost of retail drug samples in 2004 was $16 billion (Gagnon & Lexchin, 2008). Samples, in general, contribute to the rising costs of pharmaceuticals because companies want to recover their marketing expenses through higher drug prices. Also, samples encourage the use of expensive highly marketed drugs. One study found that patients who receive drug samples had higher medication expenditures than their counterparts who did not receive samples. This suggests that patients that receive samples become disproportionately burdened by drug costs (Alexander, Zhang, & Basu, 2008).

Financial need does not necessarily determine who receives samples. Based on an analysis of a large national sample, Cutrona et al. (2008) found that poor uninsured patients were *less* likely than wealthier insured patients to receive drug samples. Also, samples may impact negatively on the quality of care. This is especially true for low-income patients who cannot afford the cost of a brand name drug and/or its co-pay. For example, the medication may be discontinued when a patient finishes the "starter pack." Also samples, because they are not strictly monitored in the office setting, may be used inappropriately. Another earlier study found that drug samples were frequently dispensed to personnel and staff rather than to patients (Westfall, McCabe, & Nicholas, 1997).

Continuing education (CE)

In order to remain current about constantly evolving treatment and prescribing information, health professionals must continuously update their practice knowledge and skills. CE is one mechanism to accomplish this. Most state boards of nursing require CE credits in order to maintain licensure or prescriptive authority as do many nursing certification organizations. Conducting CE programs is expensive, and organizers may seek pharmaceutical industry support to partially or completely underwrite the costs. This support occurs in several ways including exhibit hall displays and educational grants for programs on specific topics, speaker fees, and meal symposia.

Most information that is available about industry support of CE focuses on continuing medical education (CME) for physicians. In 2007, the pharmaceutical industry spent more than 1 billion dollars to support over half of the CME programs that were provided in the United States (Accreditation Council for Continuing Medical Education, 2008). This industry practice was documented in the Institute of Medicine's (IOM) (2009b) report titled *Redesigning Continuing Education in the Health Professions*. Unfortunately, little is known about industry support of CE for APRNs. Key reports have not included information about nursing because of a notable lack of data.

While the total expenditures by industry to support CE may seem high, these programs are actually extremely profitable. One study of the return on investment for CE noted that for every $1.00 spent by the pharmaceutical industry on CE, the industry enjoys a return of $3.54 from increased prescribing of highlighted products. This return on investment is greater than the estimated cost of pharmaceutical detail visits and direct-to-consumer (DTC) advertising (Neslin, 2001). Of note, a recent report found that industry-sponsored lectures and other educational programs give more favorable treatment to a sponsor's product and tend to focus more on drug therapies than effective lifestyle modifications (American Medical Association, Council on Ethical and Judicial Affairs, 2009).

Pharmaceutical industry support of CE has been reported to effect prescribing behaviors of those that attend. One systematic review that included 10 studies of physicians found that attending industry CE events led to an increase in prescriptions of the sponsor's product (Wazana, 2000). Another study noted that CE can increase sales of a drug by promoting off-label uses (Steinman and Baron, 2007). Also, there is evidence to suggest that industry, while not overtly controlling content, can influence the educational sessions. They can suggest topics, hire lecturers, and offer grants that are consistent with the company's interests (Harrison, 2003). This may have the overall effect of shifting benefit from the patient toward that of the funder (Steinbrook, 2008). For example, industry-funded CE tends to focus more on a narrow range of topics that employ drug therapies instead of lifestyle interventions that may have a more profound lasting effect on the quality of life (Katz, Goldfinger, & Fletcher, 2002). APRN prescribers, therefore, should be aware of the potential effects that industry support may have on the content of CE programs and its potential to undermine the credibility and quality of the material presented.

The concern that commercial bias may compromise the integrity of CE in the health professions has been included in two recent IOM reports. In *Redesigning Continuing Education in the Health Professions* the IOM (2009b, p. 3) noted its concern "that some pharmaceutical and medical device companies are using continuing education inappropriately to influence health professionals so as to increase market share." Another IOM (2009a) report, *Conflict of Interest in Medical Research, Education, and Practice*, concluded that the provision of CE for healthcare professionals should undergo a broad consensus-based change that is free of industry influence.

There is mounting concern expressed by members of Congress as well. The Senate Finance Committee (2007) produced a report describing the risks of promotion-based CE. Similar to the IOM reports, the Senate report noted that drug companies often use educational grants, even those that are "unrestricted," as a way to market newer more expensive products. Furthermore, CE may be used to market products for "off-label" uses that have not been approved by the Food and Drug Administration (FDA). In 2009, the Senate Special Committee on Aging convened hearings on the commercial sponsorship of CE. Lewis Morris, the Chief Counsel, Office of the Inspector General, noted that "the current environment tolerates industry sponsors' preferential funding of programs that serve the business needs of the funders" (U.S. Senate, 2009, p. 3). This conflicts with the professional goals of both nursing and medicine that seek to direct their efforts to best serve the interest of the patient and the public good.

The controversy regarding the funding and outcomes of CE in the health professions is ongoing. One position highlights the benefit of commercial funding of CE as a legitimate mechanism for affordable and accessible CE credit. A reduction of industry support could limit professional meetings and free Internet offerings (Donnell, Marchetti, Fox, & Centor, 2009). Both the ACCME and the American Nurses Credentialing Center have instituted standards that are meant to temper industry influence on educational programs. However, auditing for industry influence on individual programs is inconsistent at best. For CME, oversight is complaint driven, occurs after the fact, and may take years to resolve (Morris, 2009). According to Steinbrook (2005, p. 535), "Given the underlying economics of CME and the small size of the ACCME [Accreditation Council for Continuing Medical Education], the goal of independence from commercial interests may be difficult to achieve."

An increasing number of educators, clinicians, and policy leaders have proposed that health professional CE move toward a system that is either free of pharmaceutical industry funding or one that employs a central funding mechanism. Industry would contribute to a central fund but could not designate that the money be spent on a specific topic or product (Brennan et al., 2006; IOM, 2009b; Josiah Macy, Jr. Foundation, 2008). However, in the absence of a central fund, some institutions have already implemented stringent guidelines to address potential conflict of interest and bias in CE programs. For example, the University of Wisconsin, which operates the largest CME program in the country, has implemented a rigorous process to prevent bias. The process includes review by a peer specially trained to identify conflict of interest in materials or presenters who are deemed to be "high risk" for industry bias (Institute of Medicine as a Profession, 2008).

Prestigious academic medical centers across the country are restricting or completely banning any kind of informational programs or lectures by medical professionals that are funded, sponsored, and/or paid for by the pharmaceutical industry in order to dispel the risk or appearance of conflicts of interest. These institutions, include, but are not limited to, Stanford University, University of Pennsylvania, University of Pittsburg, University of Michigan, University of California San Francisco, Harvard University, and Memorial Sloan-Kettering Cancer Center. The goal of this approach is to allow the healthcare professions, and especially the prescribers, to control the content and the science that is disseminated as part of their CE, without risk of bias or conflict.

Health professions are moving to recognize, mitigate, and eliminate bias in CE. APRNs should be alert to practices that can compromise the integrity of our educational offerings.

DTC marketing

DTC marketing is the advertising of pharmaceutical agents directly to consumers. To date, there are only two nations in the world that permit this type of advertising, the United States and New Zealand. DTC advertising is an addition to advertisements for drugs that were mainly directed to prescribing physicians in medical journals and through detailing. In 1985, the FDA lifted its moratorium on drug advertisements that were directed to consumers. The pharmaceutical industry quickly responded by increasing its promotional activities directed to consumers. In 1997, DTC advertising expanded when the FDA relaxed its guidelines for broadcast and electronic advertisements to the public (Suffrin & Ross, 2008). Since that time, spending by the pharmaceutical industry on DTC advertising has increased by 330%. In 2008 alone, the pharmaceutical industry spent $5 billion on this type of advertising (Donahue et al., 2007; World Health Organization, 2009).

The proliferation of DTC advertising has contributed to the evolving role of the healthcare consumer over the past several decades. Patients are no longer considered to be passive recipients of their health care and are more likely to be active participants when making clinical decisions along with their healthcare providers (Frosch, Grande, Tarn, & Kravitz, 2010; Frosch & Kaplan, 1999). The proliferation of DTC has occurred in part because of these changes, and the pharmaceutical industry has clearly taken advantage of this cultural shift.

Proponents contend that DTC advertising actively engages consumers in their care, encourages them to take their prescribed medicines by making them more aware of their diagnosis, and serves an important educational purpose (Holmer, 2002; Kelly, 2004). Moreover, one study reported that DTC advertising enhanced patient confidence when discussing health-related concerns with their physicians (Murray, Lo, Pollack, Donelan, & Lee, 2004).

Detractors note that DTC advertising results in an increase in the volume of prescriptions in general and the prescription of inappropriate medications more specifically, many times based on the desire to accommodate patients (Murray, Lo, Pollack, Donelan, & Lee, 2003; Weissman, Blumenthal, & Silk, 2004). In one study, more than half of the patients felt disappointed when they did not receive a requested medication they had seen advertised (Bell, Wilkes, Kravitz; 1999). In a survey conducted by the Kaiser Family Foundation (2008b), 44% of consumers who had asked their doctor for a prescription medication they saw on television received a prescription for the requested drug. However, it is important to note that advertisements can be confusing, especially for people with limited health literacy. In addition, the ads often lack data on cost and alternatives to medication such as lifestyle interventions (Kaphingst, Rudd, Dejong, & Daltroy, 2004; Macias, Pashupati, & Lewis, 2007; Robinson et al., 2004).

Moreover, DTC advertising can potentially expose patients to unknown risks. Typically, DTC advertisements promote drugs that have recently been released onto the market and may have unknown safety profiles. As noted above, rofecoxib (Vioxx®), Merck's blockbuster drug for arthritis, is a well-known case. It was heavily promoted by celebrities such as Dorothy Hamill in both print and television ads. Rofecoxib produced record sales for Merck before it was voluntarily withdrawn from the market when linked with excessive deaths related to cardiovascular causes (Krumholz, Ross, Pressler, & Egilman, 2007; Topol, 2004). After the withdrawal of rofecoxib, several manufacturers instituted a voluntary waiting period of 1 year after release of a medication to begin DTC ads.

PhRMA, the industry trade group, has recommended that manufacturers delay the start of advertising campaigns until prescribers have been adequately educated (PhRMA, 2005). However, it is unclear whether or not these policies on marketing have been implemented (Freudenheim, 2007). The IOM (2006) report *The Future of Drug Safety* identified potential safety issues related to new drugs. It recommended a significant restriction on drug advertising or a waiting period of at least 18 months after release for DTC advertising to occur. The FDA does not officially require a waiting period.

The FDA does, however, mandate that pharmaceutical companies disclose a "fair balance" of information in their advertisements. This includes "adequate provision" of summary information on drug indications and risks, and referral to a toll free number, website, or physician for consultation. Unfortunately, the proliferation of the DTC advertising has exceeded the monitoring capacity of regulators (Palumbo & Mullins, 2002). In November 2009, the FDA held hearings on the implications of drug advertising in emerging media such as the Internet and social networking sites. The pharmaceutical and Internet companies argued in favor of loosening rules on advertising within the context of social networking (Kuehn, 2009).

More than 60% of adults report viewing health information online, and marketers are eager to reach this audience (Pew Charitable Trust, 2009). Even without FDA regulation, this type of marketing has the potential to reach millions of consumers without oversight by the FDA. Both traditional and future advertising approaches carry the risk that information will be provided to consumers without adequate preparation to critique its quality. DTC advertising may reflect a "large and expensive uncontrolled experiment in population health" (Frosch et al., 2010, p. 24).

INDIRECT MARKETING ACTIVITIES
The medicalization of normal human experience or "disease mongering"

Direct-to-prescriber marketing strategies such as journal advertising and detailing by sales representatives are the most visible marketing methods pharmaceutical companies use to promote their products. However, there are other less visible and subtle marketing methods that can influence both the prescriber and the consumer. For example, there are a number of normal human experiences that have been medicalized to create a market for pharmaceutical interventions. As a result of this marketing, consumers may wonder if they have social anxiety disorder because they are nervous speaking to large groups, or adult attention deficit disorder because they have trouble organizing their activities for the day. The medicalization of daily life is a selling of sickness.

Medicalization is also referred to as "disease mongering," a phenomenon that has engendered increased attention over the past decade. Disease mongering is defined as the "widening of the boundaries of treatable illness in order to expand markets for those who sell and deliver treatments" (Moynihan, Heath, & Henry, 2002, p. 886). Menopause and age-related changes in erectile function are expected physiological transitions and shyness is a personality characteristic. None of these are illnesses yet they have been targeted for pharmacological treatment. In addition, minor health problems that may be self-managed are sometimes transformed into diseases requiring professional intervention such as heartburn and premenstrual mood changes (Moynihan & Henry, 2006).

Disease mongering may increase over time despite heightened awareness of its impact. In a Reuters Business Report that was directed to pharmaceutical industry executives, the author noted that "the coming years will bear greater witness to the corporate sponsored creation of disease" (Coe, 2003). Modern society is becoming increasingly dependent on quick solutions for normal human dilemmas, with a growing belief in science and innovation. This belief has been in part promoted by the proliferation of "disease awareness campaigns" designed to inform the public's understanding of disease. Many of these "educational" campaigns are underwritten by the marketing departments of pharmaceutical companies and typically encourage consumers to ask their provider about specific treatments and medications. These programs operate in tandem with marketing efforts such as drug detailing and lectures to key professional opinion leaders and DTC advertising (Burton & Rowell, 2003). Disease awareness or "educational" campaigns are used by industry to encourage consumers to discuss these conditions with their providers and request prescriptions that will alleviate the symptoms or condition.

Ghostwriting

Ghostwriting is the publication of professional journal articles that are secretly written by medical writers but purported to be officially authored by researchers. This is predominantly sponsored by pharmaceutical companies with the purpose of disseminating information favorable to a company's product (Mowatt et al., 2002). It is considered to be the unethical distribution of scientific information (LaCasse & Leo, 2010). This is a growing and troubling phenomenon that directly impacts the public's health when questionable information is disseminated for the purpose of marketing a drug (Moffatt & Elliott, 2007). For example, *The New York Times* reported that Merck staffers wrote dozens of research reports on its blockbuster drug Vioxx and paid prestigious physicians to officially author the articles, even though they were not involved in the research (Saul, 2008). A related report noted that ghostwritten articles on rofecoxib "contributed to lasting injury and even deaths as a result of prescribers and patients being misinformed about risks" (Plos Medicine Editors, 2009).

Another example of ghostwriting occurred when Wyeth hired a medical writing firm to author articles that were favorable to Premarin. These were published under the name of medical professionals who were identified as the authors. This occurred at a time when there was mounting evidence that this drug was implicated in an increased risk of breast cancer (Singer & Wilson, 2009). Recent evidence suggests that this practice continues to be a substantial problem in the medical literature and remains unabated because it is so difficult to detect (Barbour, 2010; Flanagan et al., 1998; Ross, Hill, Egilman, & Krumholtz, 2008).

To address the problem of ghostwriting, the IOM (2009a) recommended that academic medical centers prevent involvement in ghostwritten articles by professionals at their facilities. However, this practice is difficult to identify and to stop. A recent study noted that "ghost writing violates the usual norms of academia," and is considered a form of academic plagiarism (Lacasse & Leo, 2010). According to the study, only a minority (26%) of academic medical centers publicly prohibit their faculty from engaging in ghostwriting activities. As a result, the pharmaceutical industry covertly shapes the medical literature.

Promotion of medications and the effect on APRN prescribing

There has been extensive research on the effect that pharmaceutical promotion has on physicians' prescribing patterns. While there is limited empirical data on the effect of marketing on prescribing behaviors of APRNs, recent studies suggest that marketing has a similar effect on APRN prescribing as it does on physician prescribing. One study found that APRN prescribers did not believe that their interactions with representatives from industry affected their prescribing behaviors (Fischer et al., 2009). Other surveys found an uncritically positive attitude toward pharmaceutical marketing efforts (Blunt, 2004; Crigger, Barnes, Junko, Rahal, & Sheek, 2009; Jutel & Menkes, 2009; Ladd, Mahoney, & Emani, 2010). In another study, approximately half of APRN prescribers reported that they were more likely to prescribe a highlighted drug after attending an industry-sponsored meal event (Ladd et al., 2010). Another study documented high rates of prescribing of heavily promoted broad-spectrum antibiotics by nurse practitioners for viral upper respiratory tract infections (Ladd, 2005).

In recent years the pharmaceutical industry has expanded promotional efforts to APRNs. In addition to direct advertising, these activities include the same indirect techniques used to affect physician prescribing such as the creation of CE courses that contain subtle marketing messages and cultivating "key opinion leaders"— respected teachers who can appear objective while conveying promotional information (Arnold, 2004; Bacchetta & Green, 2007; Flexwell, 2005; Lee, 2006; Tarnoff, Kowalski, & Bauer, 2003).

One report by Verispan (2007), a pharmaceutical research company, noted that there was a 20% increase in marketing that was directed to APRNs in a recent 2-year period. One pharmaceutical industry trade journal reported the recent success of a national initiative called the Practicing Clinicians Exchange. The goals of the Exchange, which was underwritten by a consortium of pharmaceutical companies, was to increase representative's face time with APRNs and also to support a series of CME/CE symposia directed to APRN providers (Bacchetta & Green, 2007).

APRNs have often operated "under the radar" regarding research and educational programs that are focused on reducing nonscientific prescribing and enhancing evidence-based pharmaceutical practices. The crucial role that APRNs play in the changing landscape of health care has increased the market share of prescription drugs that they prescribe. This increase in APRN prescribing has been accompanied by an increase in drug promotions targeted at APRNs (Fortuna et al., 2008; Nazareth, Freemantle, Duggan, Mason, & Haines, 2002; Rodgers & Stough, 2007; Zwarenstein, Goldman, & Reeves, 2009). The effects of this new industry focus on APRN prescribing and on the quality of care that they provide are unknown.

While nationwide attention has focused on industry relationships with physicians, scant attention has been placed on industry relationships with APRNs. Educational and legislative efforts aimed at mitigating industry influence have focused primarily on physicians. For example, the Patient Protection and Affordable Care Act of 2010 includes "Sunshine Provisions" that require pharmaceutical and medical device manufacturers to report all payments made to *physician* prescribers for services and gifts such as consulting fees, honoraria, entertainment, food, travel, education, and research starting in 2013 (American Association of Medical Colleges, 2010). It is important to emphasize that these provisions apply only to physicians and/or teaching hospitals. The pharmaceutical industry may redirect promotional activities toward APRNs and other prescribers because of the absence of reporting constraints and no fear of legal or regulatory repercussions.

Continued promotional activities to APRNs and lack of regulatory constraints will require a new level of vigilance and ethical consideration by APRNs to assure cost-effective, evidence-based prescribing. This is especially important as practice opportunities expand with the unprecedented shortages of primary care providers.

Evidence-based prescribing

Evidence-based prescribing is the essential counterbalance to pharmaceutical industry marketing. Evidence-based prescribing has been defined as the "the conscientious, explicit, and judicious use of current best evidence in making decisions about the care of individual patients" (Sackett, Rosenberg, Gray, & Haynes, 1996, p. 71). Evidence-based prescribing is essential to the provision of quality, cost-effective care for patients.

Consequences of non-evidence-based prescribing result in the overuse and underuse of medicines, an increase in adverse reactions that lead to unnecessary hospitalizations, antimicrobial resistance, and the irrational use of medicines (British Medical Association Board of Science, 2007).

Educational strategies have been developed to encourage evidence-based prescribing by clinicians. Academic detailing is a type of prescriber education that was developed over three decades ago by a group of Harvard researchers in order to counter information that was "detailed" by industry representatives to healthcare providers. Academic detailing provides evidence-based, noncommercial information to prescribers on drugs that is disseminated with an interactive one-on-one format much like the method used by pharmaceutical detailers. This type of prescriber education has been used widely in the United States, Australia, and Canada (Markey & Schattner, 2001; Kondro, 2007). Information is disseminated in a variety of ways such as office-based visits with a provider to answer questions, newsletters, and sessions at conferences. Funding is through the government or grants, which eliminates the bias that is present when a pharmaceutical representative is attempting to sell a product (Kondro, 2007).

Research on academic detailing demonstrates that it promotes safe and appropriate drug use and has resulted in cost-effective therapeutics and adherence to evidence-based guidelines (Fretheim, Aaserud, & Oxman, 2006; O'Brien et al., 2007; Stafford et al., 2010). Academic detailing programs have been mandated in a number of states such as Massachusetts, Vermont, Minnesota, and the District of Columbia as a way to promote the judicious use of pharmaceutical therapies.

APRNs can easily implement evidence-based prescribing in their practices. First, the quality of the information that is used to make prescribing decisions should be evaluated. Critical appraisal techniques are necessary for the evaluation of the evidence. Multiple tools exist to assist providers with evaluating the findings from multiple studies. In the context of a busy clinical practice, there are readily available, evidence-based sources of information that can be accessed readily on the Internet and in print format. The following is a brief description of each resource and the methods to support evidence-based prescribing.

1. **Consumer Reports Health Best Buy Drugs (CRHBBD).** This is a nonprofit grant-funded program that publishes reports and publications on drugs based on systematic reviews of scientific research. These reviews are conducted by the Drug Effectiveness Review Project by teams of researchers. Their work undergoes an extensive peer review before publication. It is important to note that review teams have no financial interest in any pharmaceutical company or product. The reports are disseminated in formats that are designed for both consumer and prescriber audiences. There are over 22 analyses of drug classes and "CR Drug picks" are highlighted for effectiveness, cost, and safety. This information is also available in a smartphone application format. Drug information can be accessed

free of charge at http://www.consumerreports.org/health/best-buy-drugs/index.htm.

2. **Drug Effectiveness Review Project (DERP).** In response to spiraling Medicaid drug costs in Oregon, DERP was formed as a collaboration between two public entities, the Center for Evidence-Based Policy and the Oregon Evidence-Based Practice Center. The goal of DERP is to produce systematic evidence-based reviews of the safety and comparative effectiveness of common drug classes. Review teams have no financial interest in any pharmaceutical company or product. DERP reports inform numerous state Medicaid programs, in addition to the CRHBBD program, on the safety and efficacy of drugs. Information on original and updated reports is available free of charge at http://www.ohsu.edu/xd/research/centers-institutes/evidence-based-policy-center/derp/index.cfm.

3. **Independent Drug Information Service (iDiS).** The iDiS was developed by an independent group of physicians and researchers at Harvard Medical School in order to provide independent noncommercial sources of the latest information on drugs. Clinical content is developed by researchers and clinicians from Harvard Medical School who have no association with any pharmaceutical company. The program is sponsored by the Pharmaceutical Assistance Contract for the Elderly Program of the Pennsylvania Department of Aging, the Massachusetts Department of Health, and the Washington, DC Department of Health. Drug class summaries are available for professionals and consumers and are available free of charge at www.rxfacts.org.

4. **Agency for Healthcare Research and Quality (AHRQ) Effective Healthcare Program.** The Effective Healthcare Program supports research and dissemination of the comparative effectiveness of a variety of medical interventions, from surgical procedures to pharmacological therapies. It reviews, synthesizes, and compiles research findings and disseminates this information to both clinicians and consumers. Research reviews draw on completed studies in order to make "head-to-head" comparisons of treatments. They outline the benefit and/or harms of the treatments. They also publish Summary Guides that synthesize research reviews that are readily accessible for

busy clinicians. In addition, the AHRQ website offers numerous resources for clinicians and consumers, such as free, nonbiased, evidence-based CME/CE, clinician guides and social media links. See http://www.effectivehealthcare.ahrq.gov/index.cfm.

5. **The Cochrane Library.** The goal of this research group is to improve healthcare decision making globally. It uses systematic reviews and meta-analyses of the effects of healthcare interventions, including pharmaceuticals. This highly regarded resource relies solely on grants and does not accept "conflicted funding." The group supplies free clinician summaries, in a variety of languages, on many drug classes, medical conditions, and health policy issues. Their information is available free of charge at http://www.cochrane.org/.

6. *The Medical Letter/The Prescriber Letter.* These are two subscription-based sources of information that are available in print and online formats. They are both independent unbiased sources of information, especially on new drugs, and do not accept any advertisements or support from pharmaceutical companies. They are available at http://www.medicalletter.org/ and www.prescribersletter.com.

CONCLUSION

Promotional activities that are directed at prescribers and consumers are both pervasive and insidious. Pharmaceutical industry influence on prescribers is fraught with ethical issues. Many APRNs do not understand the significance of direct and indirect marketing of drugs and continue to believe they are unaffected by marketing. APRNs must increase their self-reflection, and examine their personal philosophy and institutional policies regarding interactions with drug companies and how these affect prescribing practices. Professional ethics compel us to avoid conflicts of interest that may jeopardize the high standard of care that our colleagues and patients expect.

REFERENCES

Accreditation Council for Continuing Medical Education. (2008). Annual report data, 2007. Retrieved from http://www.accme.org/dir_docs/doc_upload/207fa8e2-bdbe-47f8-9b65- 52477f9faade_uploaddocument.pdf

Adair, R., & Holmgren, L. (2005). Do drug samples influence resident prescribing behavior: A randomized trial. *The American Journal of Medicine*, *118*(8), 881–884.

Alexander, G., Zhang, J., & Basu, A. (2008). Characteristics of patients receiving pharmaceutical samples and association between sample receipt and out-of-pocket prescription costs. *Medical Care*, *46*(4), 394–402.

American Association of Medical Colleges. (2010). Physician payments sunshine provisions summary. March 2010. Retrieved from http://www.aamc.org/reform/summary/sunshine summary04022010.pdf

American Medical Association, Council on Ethical and Judicial Affairs (CEJA). (2009). CEJA report 1-A-09 financial relationships with industry in continuing education. Retrieved from http://policymed.typepad.com/files/ceja-report-on-cme-2-i-09.pdf

Arnold, M. (2004). The hidden prescribers. *Medical Marketing and Media*, *39*(11), 44.

Bacchetta, S., & Green, R. (2007). Underwriters: The importance of nurse practitioners and physician assistants. *Pharmaceutical Representative*, *37*(8), 51–61.

Barbour, V. (2010). How ghost-writing threatens the credibility of medical knowledge and medical journals. *Hematologica*, *95*(1), 1–2.

Bell, R. A., Wilkes, M. S., & Kravitz, R. L. (1999). find: Patients' anticipated reactions to a physician who refuses. *Journal of Family Practice*, *48*(6), 448–452.

Blunt, E. (2004). The influence of pharmaceutical company sponsored educational programs, promotions and gifts on the self-reported prescribing beliefs and practices of certified nurse practitioners in three states. Retrieved from http://dspace.library.drexel.edu/retrieve/3418/Blunt_Elizabeth.pdf

Boltri, J., Gordon, E., & Vogel, R. (2002). Effect of antihypertensive samples on physician prescribing patterns. *Family Medicine*, *34*(10), 729–731.

Brennan, T., Rothman, D., Blank, L., Blumenthal, D., Chimonas, S., Cohen, J., . . . Smelser, N. (2006). Health industry practices that create conflicts of interest: A policy proposal for academic medical centers. *Journal of the American Medical Association*, *295*(4), 429–433.

British Medical Association Board of Science. (2007). Evidence based prescribing. Retrieved from http://www.bma.org.uk/health_promotion_ethics/drugs_prescribing/evidencebased prescribing.jsp

Burton, B., & Rowell, A. (2003). Disease mongering. *PR Watch, 10*(1), 1–2. Retrieved from http://ics.leeds.ac.uk/papers/pmt/exhibits/2757/prwv10n1.pdf

Chew, L. D., O'Young, T. S., Hazlet, T. K., Bradley, K. A., Maynard, C., & Lessler, D. (2000). A physician survey of the effect of drug sample availability on physicians' behavior. *Journal of General Internal Medicine, 15*, 478–483.

Chimonas, S., & Kassirer, J. (2009). No more free drug samples? *PLoS Medicine, 6*(5), e1000074.

Coe, J. (2003). *Healthcare: The lifestyle drugs outlook to 2008, unlocking new value in well-being.* London: Reuters Business Insight.

Crigger, N., Barnes, K., Junko, A., Rahal, S., & Sheek, C. (2009). Nurse practitioners' perceptions and participation in pharmaceutical marketing. *Journal of Advanced Practice Nursing, 65*(3), 525–533.

Cutrona, S. L., Woolhandler, S., Lasser, K. E., Bor, D. H., McCormick, D., & Himmelstein, D. U. (2008) Characteristics of recipients of free prescription drug samples: a nationally representative analysis. *American Journal of Public Health, 98*(2):284–249.

Donahue, J., Cevasco, M., & Rosenthal, M. (2007). A decade of direct-to-consumer advertising of prescription drugs. *New England Journal of Medicine, 357*(7), 673–681.

Donnell, R., Marchetti, P., Fox, B., & Centor, R. (2009). Should we eliminate pharmaceutical funding of CME? Retrieved from http://www.medscape.com/viewarticle/586181

Fischer, M., Keough, M., Baril, J., Saccoccio, L., Mazor, K., Ladd, E., & Gurwitz, J. (2009). Prescribers and pharmaceutical representatives: Why are we still meeting? *Journal of General Internal Medicine, 24*(7), 795–801.

Flanagan, A., Carey, L., Fontanarosa, P., Phillips, S., Pace, B., Lundberg, G., & Rennie, G. (1998). Prevalence of articles with honorary authors and ghost authors in peer-reviewed medical journals. *Journal of the American Medical Association, 280*(3), 222–224.

Flexwell, N. (2005). Overlooked: Are you neglecting nurse practitioners? *Pharmaceutical Executive, 35*(3). Online publication.

Fortuna, R., Ross-Degnan, D., Finkelstein, J., Zhang, F., Campion, F., & Simon, S. (2008). Clinician attitudes towards prescribing and implications for interventions in a multi-specialty group practice. *Journal of Evaluation in Clinical Practice, 14*(6), 969–973.

Freudenheim, M. (2007). Showdown looms in congress over drug advertising on TV. The New York Times, January 22. Retrieved from: http://www.consumersunion.org/pub/pdf/Drug_Advertising_TV.pdf

Fretheim, A., Aaserud, M., & Oxman, A. (2006). Rational prescribing in primary care (RaPP): Economic evaluation of an intervention to improve professional practice. *PLoS Medicine, 3*(6), e216. doi:10.1317/journal.mned.0030216.

Frosch, D., Grande, D., Tarn, D., & Kravitz, R. (2010). A decade of controversy: Balancing policy with evidence in the regulation of prescription drug advertising. *American Journal of Public Health, 100*(1), 24–32.

Frosch, D., & Kaplan, R. (1999). Shared decision making in clinical medicine: Past research and future directions. *American Journal of Preventive Medicine, 17*(4), 285–294.

Gagnon, M., & Lexchin, J. (2008). The cost of pushing pills: A new estimate of pharmaceutical promotion expenditures in the United States. *PLoS Medicine, 5*(1), 29–33.

Greene, J. (2004). Attention to "details": Etiquette and the pharmaceutical salesman in post-war America. *Social Studies of Science, 2*, 271–292.

Greene, J. (2007). Pharmaceutical marketing research and the prescribing physician. *Annals of Internal Medicine, 46*(10), 742–748.

Harrison, R. (2003). The uncertain future of continuing medical education: Commercialism and shifts in funding. *The Journal of Continuing Education in the Health Professions, 23*(4), 198–209.

Holmer, A. (2002). Direct-to-consumer advertising: Strengthening our healthcare system. *New England Journal of Medicine, 346*(7), 526–528.

Institute of Medicine [IOM]. (2006). The future of drug safety: Promoting and protecting the health of the public. Report brief. Retrieved from http://iom.edu/Reports/2006/The-Future-of-Drug-Safety-Promoting-and-Protecting-the-Health-of-the-Public.aspx

Institute of Medicine [IOM]. (2009a). *Conflict of interest in medical research, education, and practice.* Washington, DC: National Academies Press.

Institute of Medicine [IOM]. (2009b). Redesigning continuing education in the health professions: Report Brief. Retrieved from http://iom.edu/Reports/2009/Redesigning-Continuing-Education-in-the-Health-Professions.aspx

Institute of Medicine as a Profession. (2008). Continuing medical education: Best practices for academic medical centers. Retrieved from http://www.imapny.org/File%20Library/Best%20Practice%20toolkits/CME.pdf

Jutel, A., & Menkes, D. (2009). "But doctors do it . . .": Nurse views of gifts and information from the pharmaceutical industry. *The Annals of Pharmacotherapy, 43*(6), 1057–1063.

Kaiser Family Foundation. (2008a). Prescription drug trends. Retrieved from http://www.kff.org/rxdrugs/upload/3057_07.pdf

Kaiser Family Foundation. (2008b). Public views of direct to consumer drug advertising. Retrieved from http://www.consumerreports.org/health/best-buy-drugs/index.htm

Kaphingst, K., Rudd, R., Dejong, W., & Daltroy, L. (2004). Literacy demands of product information intended to supplement television direct-to-consumer prescription drug advertisements. *Patient Education and Counseling, 55*(2), 293–300.

Katz, H., Goldfinger, S., & Fletcher, S. (2002). Academia-industry collaboration in continuing medical education: Description of two approaches. *The Journal of Continuing Education in the Health Professions, 22*(1), 43–54.

Kelly, P. (2004). DTC advertisings benefits far outweigh its imperfections. *Health Affairs,* Supplement Web Exclusives, W4-246-248.

Kondro, W. (2007). Academic drug detailing: An evidence based alternative. *Canadian Medical Association Journal, 176*(4), 429–431. doi:10.1503/cmaj.070072.

Krumholz, H., Ross, J., Pressler, A., & Egilman, D. (2007). What have we learnt from Vioxx? *British Medical Journal, 334*(7585), 120–123.

Kuehn, B. (2009). FDA weighs limits for online ads. *Journal of the American Medical Association, 303*(4), 311–313.

Lacasse, J. R., & Leo, J. (2010). Ghostwriting at elite academic medical centers in the United States. *PLoS Medicine, 7*(2), e1000230.

Ladd, E. (2005). The use of antibiotics for viral upper respiratory tract infections: An analysis of nurse practitioner and physician prescribing practices in ambulatory care, 1997–2001. *Journal of the American Academy of Nurse Practitioners, 17*(10), 416–424.

Ladd, E., Mahoney, D., & Emani, S. (2010). "Under the Radar": nurse practitioner prescribers and pharmaceutical industry promotions. *American Journal of Managed Care, 16*(12), e358–e362.

Lee, S. (2006). Invisible prescribers: What you don't know about NPs and PAs. Pharmaceutical Executive (March 1). Retrieved from http://pharmexec.findpharma.com/pharmexec/article/articleDetail.jsp?id=310978

Macias, W., Pashupati, K., & Lewis, L. (2007). A wonderful life or diarrhea and dry mouth? Policy issues of direct to consumer drug advertising on television. *Health Communications, 22*(3), 241–252.

Josiah Macy, Jr. Foundation. (2008). Chairman's summary of the conference: Continuing education in the health professions: Improving healthcare through lifelong learning. Retrieved from http://www.josiahmacyfoundation.org/documents/Macy_ContEd_1_7_08.pdf

Markey, P., & Schattner, P. (2001). Promoting evidence based medicine in general practice: The impact of academic detailing. *Family Practice, 18*(4), 364–366.

Moffatt, B., & Elliott, C. (2007). Ghost marketing: Pharmaceutical companies and ghostwritten journal articles. *Perspectives in Biology and Medicine, 50*(1), 18–31.

Morris, L. (2009). Commercial sponsorship of continuing medical education. Testimony before the Special Committee on Aging. Retrieved from http://oig.hhs.gov/testimony/docs/2009/07292009_oig_testimony.pdf

Mowatt, G., Shirran, L., Grimshaw, J., Rennie, D., Flanagin, A., Yank, V., . . . Bero, L. (2002). Prevalence of honorary and guest authorship in Cochrane reviews. *Journal of the American Medical Association, 287*(21), 2769–2761.

Moynihan, R., Heath, I., & Henry, D. (2002). Selling sickness: The pharmaceutical industry and disease mongering. *British Medical Journal*, *324*(7342), 886–891.

Moynihan, R., & Henry, D. (2006). The fight against disease mongering: Generating knowledge for action. *PLoS Medicine*, *3*(4), e191.

Murray, E., Lo, B., Pollack, L., Donelan, K., & Lee, K. (2003). Direct-to-consumer advertising: Physicians' views of its effects on quality of care and the doctor–patient relationship. *Journal of the American Board of Family Practice*, *16*(6), 513–524.

Murray, E., Lo, B., Pollack, L., Donelan, K., & Lee, K. (2004). Direct-to-consumer advertising: Public perceptions of its effects on health behaviors, health care, and the doctor–patient relationship. *Journal of the American Board of Family Practice*, *17*(1), 6–18.

Nazareth, I., Freemantle, N., Duggan, C., Mason, J., & Haines, A. (2002). Evaluation of a complex intervention for changing professional behaviour: The evidence based outreach (EBOR) trial. *Journal of Health Services Research and Policy*, *7*(4), 230–238.

Neslin, S. (2001). ROI analysis of pharmaceutical promotion(RAPP): An independent study. Retrieved from http://www.rxpromoroi.org/rapp/media/slides_speakernotes.pdf

O'Brien, M., Rogers, S., Jamtvedt, G., Oxman, A., Odgaard-Jensen, J., Kristoffersen, D., . . . Harvey, E. (2007). Educational outreach visits: Effects on professional practice and health care outcomes. *Cochrane Database of Systematic Reviews*, (4), CD000409. doi: 10.1002/14651858.CD000409.pub2.

O'Reilly, K. (2009). Doctors increasingly close doors to drug reps, while pharma cuts ranks. *American Medical News*, *52*(10). Retrieved from http://www.ama-assn.org/amednews/2009/03/23/prl10323.htm

Palumbo, F., & Mullins, C. (2002). The development of direct-to-consumer drug advertising regulation. *Food and Drug Law Journal*, *57*(3), 423–443.

Pew Charitable Trust. (2009). Internet and American life project. Retrieved from http://www.pewinternet.org/Reports/2009/8-The-Social-Life-of-Health-Information.aspx

Pharmaceutical Research and Manufacturers of America [PhRMA]. (2005). PhPRMA Guiding principles: Direct to consumer advertisements about prescription medicines. Retrieved from:

http://www.google.com/search?sourceid=navclient&ie=UTF-8 &rls=EGLC,EGLC:2007-30,EGLC:en&q=PhRMA+2005

Pharmaceutical Research and Manufacturers of America [PhRMA]. (2008). PhRMA marketing code reinforces commitment to responsible interactions with healthcare professionals. Retrieved from http://www.phrma.org/news_room/press_releases/phrma_ code_reinforces_commitment_to_responsible_interactions_ with_healthcare_professionals

Pharmaceutical Research and Manufacturers of America [PhRMA]. (2009). Code on interactions with healthcare professionals. Retrieved from http://www.phrma.org/files/attachments/ PhRMA%20Marketing%20Code%202008.pdf

Plos Medicine Editors. (2009). Ghostwriting: The dirty little secret of medical publishing that just got bigger. *PLoS Medicine, 6*(9), e1000156.

Podalsky, S., & Green, J. (2008). A historical perspective of pharmaceutical promotion and physician education. *Journal of the American Medical Association, 300*(7), 831–833.

Robinson, A., Hohmann, K., Rifkin, J., Topp, D., Gilroy, C., Pickard, J., & Anderson, R. (2004). Direct to consumer pharmaceutical advertising: Physician and public opinion and potential effects on the physician–patient relationship. *Archives of Internal Medicine, 164*(4), 427–432.

Rodgers, J., & Stough, W. (2007). Underutilization of evidence-based therapies in heart failure: The pharmacist's role. *Pharmacotherapy, 27*(4), 18S–28S.

Rosenthal, M., Berndt, E., Donahue, J., Frank, R., & Epstein, A. (2002). Promotion of prescription drugs to consumers. *New England Journal of Medicine, 346*(7), 498–505.

Ross, J., Hill, K., Egilman, D., & Krumholtz, H. (2008). Guest authorship and ghostwriting in publications related to rofecoxib: A case study of industry documents from rofecoxib litigation. *Journal of the American Medical Association, 299*(15), 1800–1812.

Sackett, J. D., Rosenberg, V. M. C., Gray, J. A. M., & Haynes, R. B. (1996). Evidence-based medicine: What it is and what it isn't. *British Medical Journal, 312*, 71–72.

Saul, S. (2008). Ghostwriters used in Vioxx studies, article says. The New York Times. April, 15, 2008.

Senate Finance Committee. (2007). Committee staff report to the chairman and ranking member: Use of educational grants by pharmaceutical manufacturers. Retrieved from http://www.arbo.org/cope/SCF%20report%20june%202005.pdf

Singer, N., & Wilson, D. (2009, September 18). Medical editors push for ghostwriting crackdown. *The New York Times*, p. B1.

Stafford, S., Bartholomew, L. K., Cushman, W., Cutler, J., Davis, B., Dawson, G., . . . & Whelton, P. (2010). Impact of ALLHAT/JNC7 dissemination project on thiazide type diuretic use. *Archives of Internal Medicine*, *170*(10), 851–858.

Steinbrook, R. (2008). Financial support of continuing medical education. *Journal of the American Medical Association*, *299*(9), 1060–1062.

Steinbrook, R. (2005). Commercial support and continuing medical education. *New England Journal of Medicine*, *352*(6), 534–535.

Steinman, M., & Baron, R. (2007). Is continuing medical education a drug promotion tool? Yes. *Canadian Family Physician*, *53*(10), 1650–1653.

Suffrin, C., & Ross, J. (2008). Pharmaceutical industry marketing: Understanding its impact on women's health. *Obstetrical and Gynecological Survey*, *63*(9), 585–596.

Tarnoff, S., Kowalski, G., & Bauer, B. (2003, May). Neglected prescribers. Pharmaceutical Sales Supplement Successful Sales Management, pp. 24–26.

Topol, E. (2004). Failing the public health: Rofecoxib, Merck, and the FDA. *New England Journal of Medicine*, *351*(17), 1707–1709.

Verispan. (2007). Personal selling audit, hospital personal selling audit, and nurse practitioner/physician assistant audit, 2004–2006. *Trends in Detail Activity*.

Wazana, A. (2000). Physicians and the pharmaceutical industry: Is a gift just a gift? *Journal of the American Medical Association*, *283*(20), 373–380.

Weissman, J., Blumenthal, D., & Silk, A. (2004). Physicians report on patient encounters involving direct-to-consumer advertising. *Health Affairs*, *W-4*(Supplement), 219–233.

Westfall, J., McCabe, J., & Nicholas, R. (1997). Personal use of drug samples by physicians and office staff. *Journal of the American Medical Association*, *278*(2), 141–143.

World Health Organization. (2009). Direct to advertising under fire. *Bulletin of the World Health Organization*, *87*(8).

Zick, C. (2009). No more free lunch: Understanding the new Massachusetts pharmaceutical and medical device marketing law and regulations. *ABA Health eSource*, *5*(12). Retrieved from http://www.abanet.org/health/esource/Volume5/12/Zick.html.

Zwarenstein, M., Goldman, J., & Reeves, S. (2009). Interprofessional collaboration: Effects of practice-based interventions on professional practice and healthcare outcomes. *Cochrane Database of Systematic Reviews*, (3), CD000072.

Regulation of Prescriptive Authority

7

Tracy Klein

This chapter provides an overview of the state and federal laws, regulations, and other factors that affect whether an advanced practice registered nurse (APRN) may prescribe autonomously. Fully autonomous prescribing is contrasted with examples of restricted prescribing authority. Discussion of the APRN Consensus Model highlights the opportunity for standardized regulation that achieves fully autonomous practice with full prescriptive authority and universal adoption of the term APRN.

Many states permit advanced practice registered nurses (APRNs) to independently assess, diagnose, and manage patients but restrict prescribing. In some states, APRNs autonomously prescribe legend[1] drugs but require some type of physician involvement to prescribe controlled substances (National Council of State Boards of Nursing [NCSBN], 2010; Pearson, 2011). Two states, Florida and Alabama, authorize nurse practitioners (NPs) to prescribe legend drugs excluding controlled substances. The remaining states authorize autonomous (independent) prescribing of both legend drugs and controlled substances.

[1] Legend drugs are any medications that require a prescription in the United States.

The Advanced Practice Registered Nurse as a Prescriber, First Edition. Marie Annette Brown, Louise Kaplan.
© 2012 John Wiley & Sons, Ltd. Published 2012 by John Wiley & Sons, Ltd.

Some states limit the controlled substances an APRN may prescribe. The majority of restrictions pertain to Schedule II drugs, which are the most controlled class of legally available drugs for patient use. Some states place other restrictions on prescribing controlled substances such as limiting the quantity that may be prescribed. States that authorize controlled substance prescribing also authorize APRNs to use individual or institutional Drug Enforcement Administration (DEA) registration (Pearson, 2011). An overview of the state and federal laws and regulations and other factors that affect whether an APRN may prescribe autonomously follows.

A MODEL FOR APRN AUTONOMOUS PRACTICE

The *Consensus Model for APRN Regulation: Licensure, Accreditation, Certification and Education* (APRN Consensus Group & the National Council of State Boards of Nursing APRN Advisory Committee, 2008) is the first fully developed model of autonomous APRN practice and is intended for national adoption. The creation of this key document is indicative of the increasing effectiveness of nursing organizations that are committed to collaboration that will benefit the profession. This was a major accomplishment for the nursing profession and serves as a foundation to create a cohesive and uniform approach to advanced practice licensure, accreditation, certification, and education (LACE). APRN practice includes the clinical nurse specialist (CNS), certified nurse practitioner (CNP), certified nurse-midwife (CNM), and certified registered nurse anesthetist (CRNA). The goal of the model is to promote recognition of autonomous practice for APRNs by licensers, accreditors, certifiers, and educators. One of the Consensus Model's foundational requirements for boards of nursing is licensing APRNs as independent practitioners with no regulatory requirements for physician collaboration, direction, or supervision (APRN Consensus Group & the National Council of State Boards of Nursing APRN Advisory Committee, 2008). Based upon this definition, in only 13 states and the District of Columbia do NPs meet the definition of being truly autonomous. As an example, Box 7.1 is the section of Washington State's rules that identifies autonomous prescribing authority. Other APRNs have less autonomy than NPs.

Box 7.1 Washington law: autonomous prescribing

WAC [Washington Administrative Code] 246-840-400
Agency filings affecting this section
ARNP prescriptive authority

(1) An ARNP licensed under chapter 18.79 RCW [Revised Code of Washington] when authorized by the nursing commission may prescribe drugs, medical equipment, and therapies pursuant to applicable state and federal laws.

(2) The ARNP, when exercising prescriptive authority, is accountable for competency in

(a) Patient selection;

(b) Problem identification through appropriate assessment;

(c) Medication or device selection;

(d) Patient education for use of therapeutics;

(e) Knowledge of interactions of therapeutics, if any;

(f) Evaluation of outcome; and

(g) Recognition and management of complications and untoward reactions.

Source: Washington Administrative Code, 2007.

Regulations for some APRN roles in various states may differ from those NPs who constitute the largest number of APRNs. Some states include certified nurse-midwives (CNMs) as NPs, for example, while others license them as a separate role or through a separate regulatory board which is the case in New York (New York State Education Department, 2009). NPs and CNMs have prescriptive authority in all 50 states and the District of Columbia. CNSs have prescriptive authority in 34 states and the District of Columbia (NCSBN, 2010). Nurse anesthetists have prescriptive authority in 28 states and the District of Columbia (Kaplan, Brown, & Simonson, 2011).

HISTORY OF APRN PRESCRIBING REGULATION

Idaho was the first state to pass prescriptive authority for NPs in 1971 (R. Hudspeth, personal communication, December 27, 2009). The law was not implemented until 1977 due to protracted requirements for joint rulemaking with the Board of Medicine (S. Evans, personal communication, December 28, 2009). Other states also authorized APRN prescriptive authority in the 1970s: Washington,

Oregon, New Mexico, Florida (CRNAs), North Carolina, Utah, and Maryland (CRNAs) (NCSBN, 2010). CNSs were often granted prescriptive authority if they specialized in psychiatry. The number of states granting prescriptive authority increased rapidly during the 1980s and 1990s (Hamric, Spross, & Hanson, 2009). However, as late as 1983, only Oregon and Washington State granted NPs and CNMs statutory autonomous prescriptive authority. Oregon's authority included Schedule III–V controlled substances. Washington's law included only Schedule V controlled substances but also extended to CRNAs.

In order to prescribe controlled substances, APRNs must register with the DEA. Not until 1993 did the DEA adopt the category "Mid-Level Provider" which permitted APRNs to register under their own unique name and number and mandated that they do so if they were prescribing controlled substances (Drug Enforcement Administration [DEA], 1993). Before 1993, registration of APRNs was done on a case-by-case basis in states which had existing autonomous prescribing authority (C. Brennan, personal communication, January 14, 2010).

During the late 1980s, CRNAs sought clarification as to whether prescribing was part of their practice. The DEA concluded that CRNAs administer medications and anesthetics in the perianesthesia period and this is considered administration or dispensing, but not prescribing (Blumenreich, 1988). APRNs who administer and dispense controlled substances as the agent of a person or facility registered with the DEA are exempt from individual registration (Blumenreich, 1993; DEA, 1993). These issues are particularly relevant to CRNAs who administer or dispense controlled substances routinely without prescriptive authority or an individual DEA registration (Blumenreich, 1993; Kaplan et al., 2011).

AUTONOMOUS PRESCRIPTIVE AUTHORITY

Autonomous prescribing is the ability to legally and independently select, prescribe, administer, dispense, and manage pharmacological treatments for individual patients regardless of setting, time frame, or circumstance. Practice barriers may restrict autonomous prescribing as significantly as legal constraints. Examples of restrictions related to APRN prescribing include:

- Requirements for a significant period of physician supervised practice (500 hours to 2 years) before prescriptive authority is granted (Maine, Colorado, California, Ohio)
- Joint jurisdiction with a medical or pharmacy board which determines scope and function of prescriptive authority or practice (North Carolina, Alabama, South Dakota, Virginia)
- Requirements to prescribe under a physician's supervision (California, Massachusetts, Minnesota, Florida, Oklahoma, Tennessee, Virginia)
- Site-based authority (Texas, Oregon for dispensing only)
- Formularies which designate in state law what may be prescribed (Ohio).

Box 7.2 shows a section of the Virginia law that requires joint jurisdiction of APRN prescribing by the Board of Nursing and Board of Medicine.

APRNs may perceive that they have autonomous prescriptive authority despite the presence of significant legal or regulatory barriers. This is sometimes true of APRNs who prescribe in states that require a collaborative or supervisory agreement with a physician only when prescribing controlled substances. These APRNs may create a practice without controlled substances or normalize this limitation and describe themselves as an autonomous prescriber. However, changes in the practice environment such as a new job can prompt them to recognize the limits that the law imposes (Kaplan, Brown, Andrilla, & Hart, 2006). Some APRNs practice without taking advantage of the legal option for autonomous prescriptive authority. Perceived barriers such as the cost of DEA registration, liability, or discomfort in changing the status quo can contribute to self-imposed limitations in prescribing (Kaplan & Brown, 2007).

Collaboration

Interprofessional collaboration need not be a barrier to autonomous prescribing and is an important aspect of comprehensive patient care (Association of Social Work Boards [ASWB] et al., 2006; Institute of Medicine [IOM], 2003). Collaborative care provided within interdisciplinary teams should be a professional norm for all health professionals in practice (IOM, 2003). In contrast,

Box 7.2 Virginia law: joint jurisdiction

§ 54.1-2957. Licensure of nurse practitioners.

The Board of Medicine and the Board of Nursing shall jointly prescribe the regulations governing the licensure of nurse practitioners.

It shall be unlawful for a person to practice as a nurse practitioner in this Commonwealth unless he holds such a joint license.

§ 54.1-2957.01. Prescription of certain controlled substances and devices by licensed nurse practitioners.

A. In accordance with the provisions of this section and pursuant to the requirements of Chapter 33 (§ 54.1-3300 et seq.) of this title, a licensed nurse practitioner, other than a certified registered nurse anesthetist, shall have the authority to prescribe controlled substances and devices as set forth in Chapter 34 (§ 54.1-3400 et seq.) of this title as follows: (1) Schedules V and VI controlled substances on and after July 1, 2000; (2) Schedules IV through VI on and after January 1, 2002; (3) Schedules III through VI controlled substances on and after July 1, 2003; and (4) Schedules II through VI on and after July 1, 2006. Nurse practitioners shall have such prescriptive authority upon the provision to the Board of Medicine and the Board of Nursing of such evidence as they may jointly require that the nurse practitioner has entered into and is, at the time of writing a prescription, a party to a written agreement with a licensed physician which provides for the direction and supervision by such physician of the prescriptive practices of the nurse practitioner. Such written agreements shall include the controlled substances the nurse practitioner is or is not authorized to prescribe and may restrict such prescriptive authority as deemed appropriate by the physician providing direction and supervision.

B. It shall be unlawful for a nurse practitioner to prescribe controlled substances or devices pursuant to this section unless such prescription is authorized by the written agreement between the licensed nurse practitioner and the licensed physician.

C. The Board of Nursing and the Board of Medicine, in consultation with the Board of Pharmacy, shall promulgate such regulations governing the prescriptive authority of nurse practitioners as are deemed reasonable and necessary to ensure an appropriate standard of care for patients.

mandatory collaboration by regulatory restriction of licensed, credentialed APRNs is widespread, and its elimination is the goal of the APRN Consensus Model. The implementation and structure of collaborative agreements vary widely from state to state. Some require that a collaborative agreement be filed with state Boards of Nursing or Boards of Medicine, while others simply mandate its presence at the practice site for review if indicated (Hanson, 2009).

In an ideal pluralistic environment, healthcare professionals would share political and economic power. Instead, organized medicine through groups such as the American Medical Association (AMA) has consistently used the legislative and regulatory processes to oppose autonomous prescribing by APRNs and exert financial and political pressure to restrict expansion of scope of practice. It is the position of the AMA (1999, 2009) that NPs, as well as all other categories of prescribers other than physicians, should not be permitted to autonomously prescribe medications. The AMA also provides funding to monitor and oppose legislation which would grant autonomous prescribing.

Lugo, O'Grady, Hodnicki, and Hanson (2007) identified factors that impact the ability of NPs to provide care and highlight how the regulatory environment affects patient access to prescription medications. Restrictive prescribing laws result in an underrepresentation of the number and type of prescriptions generated by APRNs. In states with restrictions, prescriptions are often tracked under the supervising or collaborating physician's name or DEA number. Autonomous prescribing by all APRNs is necessary to accurately determine characteristics of APRN prescribing.

The National Provider Identifier (NPI)

The National Plan and Provider Enumeration System includes a unique registration for healthcare providers known as the NPI (Department of Human Services, 2004). Prior to inception of the NPI, pharmacies often required a DEA number from prescribers for tracking purposes even if a controlled substance was not being prescribed. The NPI serves as a billing identifier for most healthcare providers regardless of their regulatory status. However, there is currently no systematic retrieval process allowing data tracking by unique NPI numbers. Nonetheless, it is strongly advised that APRN prescribers include their NPI number on prescription pads or electronic templates whether it is required by state law or individual insurance, as the number is gaining wider use and will replace Medicare billing numbers (Hanson, 2009). Use of this number also discourages inappropriate access to the DEA number for insurance billing. The NPI number could potentially be used to more accurately track APRN prescribing which could be of great benefit by demonstrating the role APRNs play in prescribing.

CONSENSUS MODEL FOR APRN REGULATION
LACE
The ability to autonomously prescribe legend drugs and controlled substances is still restricted for many APRNs despite an improved regulatory environment and the increased role of medications for therapeutic interventions with patients over the last decade. LACE refers to the four elements of APRN regulation identified in the *Consensus Model for APRN Regulation* that are essential to implementation of the model. Each element plays a unique but interdependent role in how the APRN may exercise prescriptive authority. The legal ability to prescribe pharmacological and nonpharmacological interventions is one major differentiation between the APRN and registered nurse (RN) scopes of practice according to the LACE model (APRN Consensus, 2008).

Licensing
The purpose of a regulatory licensing board is often misunderstood by the APRN. The primary purpose of a board of nursing is to protect the public. Licensing laws and requirements have been developed in the context of a libertarian theoretical perspective. This approach promotes government authority to the extent that core individual rights such as life, autonomy, and property are protected.

This context has three important implications for licensing laws. The first is the jurisdictional autonomy of each state's Board of Nursing to protect the public within that state. The second is the right of the state to determine and enforce its own laws and regulations as it sees fit (states' rights). The third is the right of the individual to legal protection against removal of private property. Both state and federal courts recognize a license as property that cannot be taken without due process (Boland, Treston, Weill, & O'Sullivan,

2009). Further, this protection is guaranteed under interpretation of the 14th Amendment and has been codified into state practice laws (Smith, 2008).

All RNs are licensed through Boards of Nursing. In a few states, APRNs still practice under joint jurisdiction with Medical Boards (NCSBN, 2010). This model was commonly used in the 1970s when prescriptive authority was new. Authority by Medical Boards of APRNs was more often imposed in relation to prescribing than other aspects of practice.

APRNs in most, but not all, states require licensure as an RN and issuance of a second license. There has been long-standing disagreement regarding the need for second licensure for APRNs (Edmunds, 1992). In August 1992, the NCSBN adopted a position paper advocating for a second license for APRN practice based upon the differences in scope of practice, including prescribing, from that of the RN (Edmunds, 1992; NCSBN, 1993). The need for a second license was opposed at that time by the American Nurses Association (ANA) based on the perspective that all nurses are under one scope of practice (Malone & Sheets, 1993). Since then, the evolution of advanced practice nursing and the accomplishments of APRNs have contributed to a deepened appreciation of APRN roles. The ANA, along with 40 other organizations, has endorsed the *Consensus Model for APRN Regulation.*

States remain divided in their approach to regulatory recognition of the APRN. Licensure is required by 47% of states for CRNAs, 51% for CNMs, 36% for CNSs, and 51% for NPs. Certification, authorization, or recognition are other regulatory mechanisms used by states (NCSBN, 2010).

In some states, prescriptive authority is granted as part of APRN licensure while in other states it is optional and requires a separate application. Prescribing authority may also require a separate designation or number, or registration with a Board of Medicine and/or Pharmacy. States with very restrictive laws, such as Michigan, do not permit APRN prescribing as part of the nurse practice act, regardless of whether a legend or controlled substance is involved. In Michigan, APRN prescribing is a delegated act under the authority of a physician (Michigan Department of Community Health, 1998–2000). The ability of Michigan NPs to prescribe is based on a 1980 state attorney general interpretation of medical laws governing physician assistants. The legal opinion added nurses to the category of health professionals to whom a physician can delegate prescribing of legend drugs, excluding controlled substances (Michigan Department, 1980).

The ability to obtain prescriptive authority, whether restricted, optional, or mandatory, usually involves specific requirements (Hanson, 2009; NCSBN, 2010). These include a minimum number of hours of pharmacology in the original educational program, pharmacotherapeutics continuing education (CE), collaborative agreements, and additional state prescribing licenses or DEA registration (Hanson, 2009).

Some states do not permit autonomous or even collaborative prescriptive authority under the APRN's own license until completion of a supervised period of prescribing practice. For example, Maine requires 2 years of supervised practice including prescribing before autonomous prescriptive authority is issued (Pearson, 2011). Colorado requires 3600 hours of independent prescribing in another state or an 1800-hour "mentorship" with a physician or a physician and advanced practice nurse with prescriptive authority. Prescriptive authority under a collaborative practice arrangement can then be authorized for NPs (Colorado Board of Nursing, 2010).

Accreditation
APRN programs are accredited by degree or role. Master's in nursing and Doctor of Nursing Practice programs are accredited by the National League for Nursing Accreditation Commission or the Commission on Collegiate Nursing Education (CCNE). Nurse-midwifery and nurse anesthetist programs are additionally accredited through the Accreditation Commission for Midwifery Education (ACME) and the Council on Accreditation (COA) of Nurse Anesthesia programs, respectively.[2]

Standards and competencies for NPs developed by the National Organization of Nurse Practitioner Faculties (NONPF) are incorporated into the CCNE accreditation process of NP programs (National Task Force, 2008). To insure quality education, NONPF's core competencies for NP practice are used to develop curriculum

---

[2] APRN programs that are not in schools of nursing may only have ACME or COA accreditation.

and student outcomes. There is only one core competency related to prescribing.

Only one major nursing organization, the ANA, has published a standard of care regarding prescribing. Standard 5D of ANA's (2010) *Nursing: Scope and Standards of Practice* establishes a standard and a set of competencies for APRN prescriptive authority. None of the national associations for CNMs, CRNAs, and CNSs has standards that address prescribing competencies specifically (Klein & Kaplan, 2010).

APRN accreditation standards generally set criteria for pharmacology coursework. Educational programs determine how the course is applied in the curriculum and which components of state and federal prescribing laws to include. In addition to an advanced pharmacology course, pharmacological principles are integrated across the educational program and clinical practica. The APRN student graduates with the ability to manage patients using pharmacological therapy.

Certification

National certifying exams are developed by the professions to validate role, specialty, or population-specific competencies. APRN certification examinations validate entry-level knowledge and abilities for practice (Chornick, 2008). The majority of states require national certification for initial APRN licensure as well as maintenance of licensure (NCSBN, 2010). National certification has been required for CRNAs in order to qualify for Medicare reimbursement since 1992 (U.S. Code of Federal Regulations, 2008). In 2003, the Center for Medicare and Medicaid Services (CMS) required national certification for first-time NP, CNM, and CNS applicants (U.S. Code of Federal Regulations, 2008). Many state and private insurers also require national certification for credentialing.

National certification exams are based upon job analysis and role delineation studies that are updated periodically. As the number of APRNs with prescriptive authority and autonomous practice increases, future job analysis studies and the content of national certification exams may be affected. At this time, the prescriber role, though integral to the APRN practice, is a small component of national certification examinations. For example, pharmacological and prescribing content that is covered in the American Nurses

Credentialing Center family NP certification examination includes questions related to pharmacology, pharmacotherapeutics management, electronic prescribing, and use of non-pharmacological or complementary therapies (American Nurses Credentialing Center, 2009). National certification examinations do not test specifics of state law and requirements for prescribing. State-specific prescribing competencies should be included in the basic educational preparation for APRNs as well as incorporated into their ongoing licensure renewal requirements.

Education

Licensure, accreditation, and certification contribute to the educational design of curricula and preparation of APRNs as prescribers. Changes in education based on regional needs and evolution of APRN roles could contribute to enhanced prescriptive competencies (ASWB et al., 2006). Even when state restrictions exist, all APRNs should be educated for autonomous practice to facilitate professional mobility (Klein & Kaplan, 2010). National consensus documents can help guide curricular design for pharmacology courses in APRN programs (Yocum, Busby, Conway-Welch, & Viens, 1999).

NP and CRNA eligibility for national certification requires that the educational program verify completion of a minimum of three credits of graduate-level pharmacology. This requirement is consistent with the American Association of Colleges of Nursing's standards for doctoral and master's programs that prepare nurses for advanced practice. Educational programs should document through course descriptions, transcripts, and curricular materials the specific competencies necessary for prescriptive authority as they are developed throughout the curriculum and clinical practica (Klein & Kaplan, 2010).

It is also the responsibility of educators to assure graduates are eligible for national certification and state licensure (APRN Consensus, 2008). Distance learning programs and multiple campus delivery technology blur the boundaries of state-based education, increasing the responsibility of the student to carefully evaluate prescribing laws in the state where he or she will practice. Additionally, the ability to prescribe may not be available for a CRNA or a CNS in their chosen state of practice. This may create a need for additional education when the law changes to permit prescribing for the first time or when an APRN moves to another state and desires to apply for this authority (Klein & Kaplan, 2010).

There may also be educational requirements, in addition to those in the initial program, when an APRN wants to reactivate licensure after a period of not practicing or prescribing. Reentry requirements for APRNs are developed on a state-by-state basis. Oregon, as an example, requires that an NP demonstrate at least 400 hours of utilizing pharmacological knowledge in order to renew licensure and prescriptive authority (Oregon State Board of Nursing, 2007). Failure to do so requires completion of a 45-hour pharmacology course (Oregon State Nurse Practice Act, 2009) and may also require an additional prescribing practicum.

Prescriptive authority renewal requirements for prescribing in some states may be met through CE courses. These may be offered by academic institutions, nonprofit organizations, or for-profit CE companies. It is important to verify directly with the licensing board and national certifying organization which courses may be used toward renewal requirements. Boards and national certifying bodies generally accept nursing, pharmacy, or medical accreditation for pharmacology and prescribing courses. Common accrediting bodies include the Accreditation Council for Pharmacy Education, the Accreditation Council for Medical Education, and the American Nurses Credentialing Center.

OTHER REGULATORY REQUIREMENTS

APRNs may now be credentialed by healthcare systems as licensed independent practitioners under the Joint Commission guidelines adopted in their ambulatory care manual (Joint Commission on Accreditation of Healthcare Organizations, 2004). In states where autonomous practice is legally permitted, facilities may credential an APRN to admit, discharge, manage, and prescribe for patients on an inpatient or outpatient basis. There is limited legal or regulatory guidance regarding credentialing to practice within a facility (Klein, 2008). When credentialing, a facility may limit prescribing or restrict an APRN's legal scope of practice but may not broaden it beyond state and federal law.

Federal agencies such as the Veterans Administration (VA), may also credential an APRN to prescribe. These agencies require the APRN to have state licensure (not necessarily in the state of practice), national certification, a master's or doctoral degree, and completion of a graduate-level course in pharmacology (Department of Veterans Affairs, 2008). As an example, an NP prescribing in a Tennessee VA hospital may prescribe autonomously under her Oregon license if credentialed by the VA even though Tennessee law requires physician supervision.

PRESCRIPTIVE AUTHORITY LIMITATIONS

There are many types of limitation to prescriptive authority, not all of which are legally imposed. It is important for APRNs to understand the source of a prescribing limit in order to effect change. Limits to prescribing for APRNs may originate in law, regulation, policy, or custom. Some limits to prescribing apply specifically to controlled substances and apply to all prescribers, not just APRNs (see Box 7.3). Another example of a limitation pertains to federally registered methadone treatment centers that are prohibited from treating opioid addiction with any medication other than methadone. Similarly, the Drug Addiction Treatment Act (2000) allows only physicians to prescribe and dispense buprenorphine for treatment of opioid addiction in an office setting.

Some prescribing limits have their foundation in safety, efficacy, cost, availability, or patient-specific indications. For example, an insurer may limit coverage of a medication to its standardized dosing parameters for the average individual patient or limit the number of pills that are a covered benefit each month. The Food and Drug Administration may require that a drug be prescribed as part of a "limited access program" to specific patient populations such as people with a specific type of cancer and treatment response. Other limits, such as those restricting prescribing of controlled substance to a 72-hour supply, are unnecessary and negatively impact APRN practice and patient access to care. The safe prescriber self-evaluates to identify limits to prescribing in accordance with scope of practice, knowledge, competency, and evidence. A discussion of specific strategies to address and remove prescribing limitations can be found in Chapter 3.

Box 7.3 Utah controlled substance act: applies to all prescribers

R156-37-603. Restrictions Upon the Prescription, Dispensing and Administration of Controlled Substances.

(1) A practitioner may prescribe or administer the Schedule II controlled substance cocaine hydrochloride only as a topical anesthetic for mucous membranes in surgical situations in which it is properly indicated and as local anesthetic for the repair of facial and pediatric lacerations when the controlled substance is mixed and dispensed by a registered pharmacist in the proper formulation and dosage.

(2) A practitioner shall not prescribe or administer a controlled substance without taking into account the drug's potential for abuse, the possibility the drug may lead to dependence, the possibility the patient will obtain the drug for a nontherapeutic use or to distribute to others, and the possibility of an illicit market for the drug.

(3) When writing a prescription for a controlled substance, each prescription shall contain only one controlled substance per prescription form and no other legend drug or prescription item shall be included on that form.

(4) In accordance with Subsection 58-37-6(7)(f)(v)(D), unless the prescriber determines there is a valid medical reason to allow an earlier dispensing date, the dispensing date of a second or third prescription shall be no less than 30 days from the dispensing date of the previous prescription, to allow for receipt of the subsequent prescription before the previous prescription runs out.

(5) If a practitioner fails to document his intentions relative to refills of controlled substances in Schedules III through V on a prescription form, it shall mean no refills are authorized. No refill is permitted on a prescription for a Schedule II controlled substance.

(6) Refills of controlled substance prescriptions shall be permitted for the period from the original date of the prescription as follows:
  (a) Schedules III and IV for 6 months from the original date of the prescription; and
  (b) Schedule V for 1 year from the original date of the prescription.

(7) No refill may be dispensed until such time has passed since the date of the last dispensing that 80% of the medication in the previous dispensing should have been consumed if taken according to the prescriber's instruction.

Continued

(8) No prescription for a controlled substance shall be issued or dispensed without specific instructions from the prescriber on how and when the drug is to be used.

(9) Refills after expiration of the original prescription term requires the issuance of a new prescription by the prescribing practitioner.

(10) Each prescription for a controlled substance and the number of refills authorized shall be documented in the patient records by the prescribing practitioner.

(11) A practitioner shall not prescribe or administer a Schedule II controlled stimulant for any purpose except

   (a) the treatment of narcolepsy as confirmed by neurological evaluation;

   (b) the treatment of abnormal behavioral syndrome, attention deficit disorder, hyperkinetic syndrome, or related disorders;

   (c) the treatment of drug-induced brain dysfunction;

   (d) the differential diagnostic psychiatric evaluation of depression;

   (e) the treatment of depression shown to be refractory to other therapeutic modalities, including pharmacological approaches, such as tricyclic antidepressants or MAO inhibitors;

   (f) in the terminal stages of disease, as adjunctive therapy in the treatment of chronic severe pain or chronic severe pain accompanied by depression;

   (g) the clinical investigation of the effects of the drugs, in which case the practitioner shall submit to the division a written investigative protocol for its review and approval before the investigation has begun. The investigation shall be conducted in strict compliance with the investigative protocol, and the practitioner shall, within 60 days following the conclusion of the investigation, submit to the division a written report detailing the findings and conclusions of the investigation; or

   (h) in treatment of depression associated with medical illness after due consideration of other therapeutic modalities.

Medication samples

Many nurse practice acts specifically include language regarding the APRNs' ability to receive, distribute, and sign for samples as part of their prescriptive authority. The Prescription Drug Marketing Act (PDMA) of 1987 was intended to address drug diversion and sales of samples by providing regulations to track their distribution (Angarola & Beach, 1996; Food and Drug

Administration, 2009; Romanski, 2003). Implementation of the law in 2000, however, resulted in many APRNs being denied the ability to sign for or receive samples without a supervising physician signature. There was confusion about prescribing requirements among drug companies who found it difficult to review and evaluate APRN prescribing laws state by state. Many developed forms that defaulted to the strictest state laws requiring physician supervision and a physician signature for samples.

APRNs in some states successfully challenged this interpretation of the PDMA. Other APRN professional groups, such as those in California, were able to use the confusion of the PDMA to pass laws explicitly permitting receipt of samples for NPs, replacing laws that had been unclear or prohibitive (California Board of Registered Nursing, 2000; Phillips, 2002).

Formularies

Some Boards of Nursing, when required by law, adopted formularies for APRN prescribing. A formulary is a list of drugs, drug classes, or drug categories that may be prescribed by health professionals within the scope of their licensure. Many formularies required approval by physicians and/or pharmacists, from nurse prescribers. States such as Oregon and New Hampshire adopted formularies as a compromise to enable other aspects of autonomous practice (Pruitt, Wetsel, Smith, & Spitler, 2002). Once adopted, formularies can take many years to remove. Oregon's formulary requirement was removed in 2008 after 29 years (State of Oregon, 2008) while the New Hampshire formulary requirement was removed in 2009 after 25 years (Sampson, 2009; State of New Hampshire, 2009).

Dispensing

The DEA (2007) defines dispensing as follows:

> The term "dispense" means to deliver a controlled substance to an ultimate user or research subject by, or pursuant to the lawful order of, a practitioner, including the prescribing and administering of a controlled substance and the packaging, labeling or compounding necessary to prepare the substance for such delivery. The term "dispenser" means a practitioner who so delivers a controlled substance to an ultimate user or research subject."

State law that defines dispensing may be more restrictive than the federal definition. Box 7.4 defines Oregon dispensing law for nurses with prescriptive authority. Broader dispensing authority is primarily accorded to physicians, pharmacists, and veterinarians. The ability to apply for and be granted dispensing authority varies greatly for APRNs from state to state. APRNs have been subject in state law to limitations on their dispensing authority as well as their ability to distribute samples. Examples of dispensing restrictions may include geographic location, ability to charge or bill, quantity, type of medication, and patient population.

The distribution of samples to a patient is not defined as "dispensing" in accordance with federal law (Code of Federal Regulations, 2008). States often exclude sample distribution from dispensing law. Oregon pharmacy law, for example, defines distribution as "the delivery of a drug other than by administering or dispensing" (Oregon Revised Statute, 2007c). Distribution includes samples that are given to patients by an APRN who lacks dispensing authority (Oregon Revised Statute, 2007a, 2007b). APRNs who dispense medications may be required to obtain a separate dispensing license and meet specific criteria. Alternately, dispensing authority may be included as part of prescriptive authority. In addition, some states mandate dispensing limits for controlled substances. Kentucky, for example, completely prohibits dispensing of controlled substances (Kentucky Board of Nursing, 2011).

Quantity limitations

The quantity of medications prescribed or dispensed by APRNs, especially controlled substances, are sometimes limited by state law. A search of the literature revealed no evidence that a restriction in the amount of medication prescribed or dispensed by APRNs is necessary to assure APRNs offer quality care. Presumably, these restrictions are part of the effort by organized medicine to limit APRN practice (AMA, 2009). Nonetheless, Kentucky limits the prescribing of controlled substances to a 72-hour supply for Schedule II medications. An exception is made for mental health APRNs who prescribe psychostimulants in specific settings (Kentucky Revised Statute, 2007). Quantity limitations for controlled substances are also found in state law in Montana (48-hour supply), Nebraska (72-hour supply), Ohio (72-hour supply),

Box 7.4 Oregon law: dispensing limits

678.390 Authority of nurse practitioner and clinical nurse specialist to write prescriptions or dispense drugs; notice; requirements; revocation; rules.

(1) The Oregon State Board of Nursing may grant to a certified nurse practitioner or certified clinical nurse specialist the privilege of writing prescriptions described in the formulary under ORS 678.385.

(2) A certified nurse practitioner or certified clinical nurse specialist may submit an application to the Oregon State Board of Nursing to dispense prescription drugs. The Oregon State Board of Nursing shall provide immediate notice to the State Board of Pharmacy upon receipt and upon approval of an application from a certified nurse practitioner or certified clinical nurse specialist for authority to dispense prescription drugs to the patients of the applicant.

(3) An application for the authority to dispense prescription drugs as authorized under subsection (1) of this section must include:

    (a) Evidence of completion of a prescription drug dispensing training program jointly developed and adopted by rule by the Oregon State Board of Nursing and the State Board of Pharmacy.

    (b) Except when a certified nurse practitioner is seeking authority to dispense prescription drugs at a qualified institution of higher education as defined in ORS 399.245, demonstration of a lack of readily available access to pharmacy services in the practice area of the applicant and that the lack of access would be corrected by granting authority to dispense prescription drugs by the applicant. Lack of readily available access to pharmacy services for patients may be established by evidence:

        (A) That the patients of the applicant are located

            (i) Outside the boundaries of a metropolitan statistical area;

            (ii) Thirty or more highway miles from the closest hospital within the major population center in a metropolitan statistical area; or

            (iii) In a county with a population of less than 75,000.

        (B) Of financial barrier to access, including but not limited to receiving services from a healthcare safety net clinic or eligibility for participation in a patient assistance program of a pharmaceutical company.

    (c) Any other information required by the Oregon State Board of Nursing.

Pennsylvania (72-hour supply), and Texas (30-day supply) (DEA, 2010).

Co-signatures

States with supervision or collaborative agreements do not require a physician to co-sign prescriptions. An APRN with prescriptive authority for a class of drugs may sign her own prescription unless the collaborative agreement stipulates that the physician must also sign (Byrne, 2009). In other situations, a physician must write the prescription for a patient when the NP does not have prescriptive authority for drugs such as controlled substances.

Designation of the responsible prescriber

There have been recent changes to laws that address what provider information is required on prescriptions. In 2004, for example, NPs in California successfully passed legislation that required including an NP's name along with the physician supervisor's on both the prescription and the medication's label (California State Senate, 2004). The lack of the NP's name on medication labels rendered NPs invisible in the prescribing aspect of patient care. Many states do, however, require that both the NP's and collaborating or supervising physician's name and address be printed on a prescription pad or label when an APRN is the prescriber (Byrne, 2009).

Mail order/prescribing across state lines

The ability to fill a prescription written by an APRN from another state is either specifically permitted or at the pharmacist's discretion in accordance with state pharmacy law. It is increasingly more common for insurers to encourage use of mail-order pharmacies causing confusion regarding APRN prescribing authority. NP Harriet Hellman (2002) testified before the Federal Trade Commission regarding problems experienced by some patients of NPs when mail-order pharmacies delayed filling or refused legitimate prescriptions. The adoption of uniform and consistent requirements for APRN prescribing would reduce this type of confusion.

CONCLUSION

APRN authority to prescribe varies greatly from state to state and among APRN roles. Disparities among national APRN regulations related to prescribing reflect diverse sociocultural and political norms and may affect the professional development of the APRN prescriber. National adoption of the APRN Consensus Model is necessary to eliminate these disparities. Evidence-based prescribing competencies can also be used to develop uniform regulatory requirements. The ultimate goal is to create the opportunity for APRNs to practice to the full scope of their expertise and to establish autonomous prescribing authority for all APRNs (Klein & Kaplan, 2010).

REFERENCES

American Medical Association. (1999). Report of the council on medical service. Non-Physician prescribing. Resolution 511, A-98. Author.

American Medical Association. (2009). *AMA scope of practice data series: Nurse practitioners*. Chicago, IL: Author. Retrieved from http://www.acnpweb.org/files/public/08-0424_SOP_Nurse_Revised_10_09.pdf

American Nurses Association. (2010). *Nursing: Scope and standards of practice*. Silver Spring, MD: Author.

American Nurses Credentialing Center. (2009). Family nurse practitioner board certification test content outline: Effective date March 1, 2010. Retrieved from http://www.nursecredentialing.org/Documents/Certification/TestContentOutlines/FamilyNPMar2010.aspx

Angarola, R., & Beach, J. (1996). The prescription drug marketing act: A solution in search of a problem? *Food and Drug Law Journal*, *51*(1), 21–55.

APRN Consensus Group & the National Council of State Boards of Nursing APRN Advisory Committee. (2008). Consensus model for APRN regulation: licensure, accreditation, certification & education.

Association of Social Work Boards [ASWB], Federation of State Boards of Physical Therapy, Federation of State Medical Boards, National Association of Boards of Pharmacy, National Board for Certification in Occupational Therapy, & National Council of State Boards of Nursing. (2006). Changes in healthcare professions' scope of practice: Legislative considerations. Retrieved from https://www.ncsbn.org/ScopeofPractice.pdf

Blumenreich, G. A. (1988). Nurse anesthetists and prescriptive authority. *The Journal of the American Association of Nurse Anesthetists, 56*(2), 91–93.

Blumenreich, G. A. (1993). Legal briefs: Drug enforcement administration mid-level practitioner regulation. Retrieved from http://www.aana.com/Resources.aspx?id=2409#Summary%20of%20Drug

Boland, B., Treston, J., Weill, V., & O'Sullivan, A. (2009). Are you ready for the consensus model? Implications of the model act on NP practice. *The American Journal for Nurse Practitioners, 13*(11/12), 10–21.

Byrne, W. (2009). US nurse practitioner prescribing law. Retrieved from http://www.medscape.com/viewarticle/440315

California Board of Registered Nursing. (2000). Nurse practitioners new authority to provide medications. Retrieved from www.rn.ca.gov/pdfs/regulations/npr-b-26.pdf.

California State Senate. (2004). AB 2660. Retrieved from http://info.sen.ca.gov/cgi-bin/postquery

Chornick, N. (2008). APRN licensure versus APRN certification: what is the difference? *JONAS Healthcare Law Ethics and Regulation, 10*(4), 90–93.

Code of Federal Regulations. (2008). 21 CFR Part 208- Medication guides for prescription drug products. S208.3. Retrieved from http://ecfr.gpoaccess.gov/cgi/t/text/text-idx?c=ecfr&tpl=/ecfrbrowse/Title21/21cfr208_main_02.tpl

Colorado Board of Nursing. (2010). Rules and regulations regarding prescriptive authority for advanced practice nurses. Retrieved from http://www.dora.state.co.us/nursing/rules/ChapterXVRevisionsFinalposthearing.pdf

Department of Human Services. (2004). HIPAA administrative simplification: Standard unique health identifier for health care providers. Final Rule, 45 CFR Part 162. Retrieved from http://www.cms.hhs.gov/NationalProvIdentStand/Downloads/NPIfinalrule.pdf

Department of Veterans Affairs. (2008). Establishing medication prescribing authority for advanced practice nurses. VHA Directive 2008-49. Retrieved from http://www1.va.gov/VHAPUBLICATIONS/ViewPublication.asp?pub_ID=1746

Drug Addiction Treatment Act. (2000). Public law 106-310-106th congress. Retrieved from http://www.buprenorphine.samhsa.gov/fulllaw.html

Drug Enforcement Administration. (1993). Definition and registration of mid-level providers, 58 FR 31907.

Drug Enforcement Administration. (2007). Title 21 United States Code (USC) controlled substances act section 802. Definitions. Retrieved from http://www.deadiversion.usdoj.gov/21cfr/21usc/802.htm

Drug Enforcement Administration. (2010). Mid-level practitioners authorization by state. Retrieved from http://www.deadiversion.usdoj.gov/drugreg/practioners/mlp_by_state.pdf

Edmunds, M. (1992). Council's pursuit of national standardization for advanced practice nursing meets with resistance. *The Nurse Practitioner*, *17*(10), 81–83.

Food and Drug Administration. (2009). Prescription drug marketing act of 1987. Retrieved from http://www.fda.gov/RegulatoryInformation/Legislation/FederalFoodDrugandCosmeticActFDCAct/SignificantAmendmentstotheFDCAct/PrescriptionDrugMarketingActof1987/default.htm

Hamric, A. B., Spross, J. A., & Hanson, C. M. (Eds.). (2009). *Advanced practice nursing: An integrative approach* (4th ed.). St. Louis, MO: Elsevier.

Hanson, C. (2009). Understanding regulatory, legal, and credentialing requirements. In A. B. Hamric, J. A. Spross, & C. M. Hanson (Eds.), *Advanced practice nursing: An integrative approach* (4th ed.). St. Louis, MO: Elsevier.

Hellman, H. (2002, October 9). The impact on consumers of possible anticompetitive efforts to restrict competition on the internet: Telemedicine and pharmaceutical online sales. Testimony to the Federal Trade Commission. Retrieved from http://www.ftc.gov/opp/ecommerce/anticompetitive/panel/hellman.pdf

Institute of Medicine [IOM]. (2003). *Health professions education: A bridge to quality*. Washington, DC: National Academies Press.

Joint Commission on Accreditation of Healthcare Organizations. (2004). *The Medical Staff Handbook: A Guide to Joint Commission Standards* (2nd ed.). Oakbrook Terrace, IL: Joint Commission on Accreditation of Healthcare Organizations.

Kaplan, L., & Brown, M. A. (2007). The transition of nurse practitioners to changes in prescriptive authority. *Journal of Nursing Scholarship, 39*(2), 184–190.

Kaplan, L., Brown, M. A., Andrilla, H., & Hart, L. G. (2006). Barriers to autonomous practice. *Nurse Practitioner, 31*(1), 57–63.

Kaplan, L., Brown, M. A., & Simonson, D. C. (2011). CRNA prescribing practices: The Washington state experience. *AANA Journal, 79*(1), 24–29.

Kentucky Board of Nursing. (2011). APRN practice. Retrieved from http://kbn.ky.gov/practice/aprn_practice.htm

Kentucky Revised Statute. (2007). KRS 314.011(8). Retrieved from http://www.lrc.ky.gov/KRS/314-00/011.PDF

Klein, T. (2008). Credentialing the nurse practitioner in your workplace. *Nursing Administration Quarterly, 32*(4), 273–278.

Klein, T., & Kaplan, L. (2010). Prescribing competencies for advanced practice registered nurses. *The Journal for Nurse Practitioners, 6*(2), 115–122.

Lugo, N., O'Grady, E., Hodnicki, D., & Hanson, C. (2007). Ranking state NP regulation: Practice environment and consumer healthcare choice. *The American Journal for Nurse Practitioners, 11*(4), 8–24.

Malone, B., & Sheets, V. (1993). Second licensure? ANA and NCSBN debate the issue. *The American Nurse, 25*(8), 8–9.

Medical Practice Act of the Code of Virginia. (2007). Chapter 29. Medicine and other healing arts. Retrieved from http://www.dhp.virginia.gov/nursing/nursing_laws_regs.htm

Michigan Department of Community Health. (1998–2000). Delegation of prescribing of controlled substances to nurse practitioners or nurse midwives: Limitations. R 338.2305. Retrieved from http://www.state.mi.us/orr/emi/admincode.asp?AdminCode=Department&Dpt=CH&Level_1=Bureau+of+Health+Professions

Michigan Department of the Attorney General. (1980). Prescriptions by a nurse or physician's assistant. Opinion no. 5630. Retrieved from http://www.ag.state.mi.us/opinion/datafiles/1980s/op05630.htm

National Council of State Boards of Nursing. (1993). Regulation of advanced nursing practice: NCSBN position paper, 1993. Retrieved from https://www.ncsbn.org/1993_Position_Paper_on_the_Regulation_of_Advanced_Nursing_Practice.pdf

National Council of State Boards of Nursing. (2010). Member Board Profiles. Retrieved from https://www.ncsbn.org/2010_Regulation_of_Advanced_Practice_Nursing.pdf

National Task Force on Quality Nurse Practitioner Education. (2008). *Criteria for evaluation of nurse practitioner programs.* Washington, DC: National Organization of Nurse Practitioner Faculties.

New York State Education Department. (2009). Regulations of the commissioner. Subpart 79-5.6. Retrieved from http://www.op.nysed.gov/prof/midwife/part79-5.htm#pres

Oregon Revised Statutes. (2007a). Authority of nurse practitioner and clinical nurse specialist to write prescriptions or dispense drugs; notice; requirements; revocation; rules. Retrieved from http://www.leg.state.or.us/ors/678.html

Oregon Revised Statutes. (2007b). Nurse practitioners; certificates; prohibitions; authority to sign death certificates; drug prescriptions. Retrieved from http://www.leg.state.or.us/ors/678.html

Oregon Revised Statutes. (2007c). Pharmacists; drug outlets; drug sales; occupations and professions; general provisions. Retrieved from http://landru.leg.state.or.us/ors/689.html

Oregon State Board of Nursing. (2007). Policy guideline: Utilization of prescriptive authority for clinical nurse specialists and nurse practitioners. Retrieved from http://www.oregon.gov/OSBN/pdfs/policies/prescribing.pdf

Oregon State Nurse Practice Act. (2009). Division 56. Retrieved from www.oregon.gov/OSBN

Pearson, L. (2011). The Pearson report. Retrieved from http://www.pearsonreport.com/

Phillips, S. J. (2002). California NPs claim pharmaceutical victory. *Nurse Practitioner, 27*(10), 25.

Pruitt, R., Wetsel, M. A., Smith, K., & Spitler, H. (2002). How do we pass NP autonomy legislation? *The Nurse Practitioner, 27*(3), 56–65.

Romanski, J. (2003). The final sampling regulations of the prescription drug monitoring act are alive and well: Is your sampling program compliant? *Food and Drug Law Journal, 58*(4), 649–660.

Sampson, D. (2009). Alliances of cooperation: Negotiating New Hampshire nurse practitioners' prescribing practice. *Nursing History Review, 17*(1), 153–178.

Smith, M. (2008). Legal basics for professional nursing: Nurse practice acts. *Center for American Nurses Continuing Education*. Retrieved from http://www.nursingworld.org/mods/mod995/print.pdf

State of New Hampshire. (2009). SB 66, Chapter 54 Stat. Ann. Retrieved from http://www.gencourt.state.nh.us/legislation/2009/SB0066.html

State of Oregon. (2008). SB 1062, ORS 678.375, Section 2, Stat. Ann. Retrieved from http://www.leg.state.or.us/08ss1/measpdf/sb1000.dir/sb1062.en.pdf

U.S. Code of Federal Regulations. (2008). Services of a certified registered nurse anesthetist or an anesthesiologist's assistant: Basic rule and definitions; nurse practitioner services, clinical nurse specialist services. CFR 410.7569-76. Retrieved from http://edocket.access.gpo.gov/cfr_2007/octqtr/pdf/42cfr410.75.pdf

Utah Controlled Substances Act Rules. (2008). Restrictions upon the prescription, dispensing and administration of controlled substances. R156-37-603. Retrieved from http://statelicenseservicing.com/files/R156-37.pdf

Washington Administrative Code 246-840-400. (2007) ARNP prescriptive authority. Retrieved from http://apps.leg.wa.gov/WAC/default.aspx?cite=246-840-400

Yocum, C., Busby, L., Conway-Welch, C., & Viens, D. (1999). Curriculum guidelines and regulatory criteria for family nurse practitioners seeking prescriptive authority to manage pharmacotherapeutics in primary care: Summary Report 1998. National Council of State Boards of Nursing and National Organization of Nurse Practitioner Faculties.

Legal Aspects of Prescribing

Carolyn Buppert

This chapter reviews key legal information to help advanced practice registered nurses avoid missteps with the prescriber role. The exemplars highlight the role of Boards of Nursing, malpractice attorneys when a lawsuit is filed, the Drug Enforcement Administration, and government auditors who monitor nursing facilities.

What do advanced practice registered nurses (APRNs) who prescribe medications need to know about the law?

- First, they need to know what authority they have under state law and the state's legal requirements for prescribing.
- Second, they need to know the federal laws on prescribing controlled substances.
- Third, they need to know the standard of care for prescribing the classes of drugs they intend to prescribe.

It is instructive to review situations that have resulted in legal action against APRNs. In addition to peer review by colleagues, there are four entities that have the authority to scrutinize prescribing practices of APRNs. These are Boards of Nursing, malpractice

The Advanced Practice Registered Nurse as a Prescriber, First Edition. Marie Annette Brown, Louise Kaplan.
© 2012 John Wiley & Sons, Ltd. Published 2012 by John Wiley & Sons, Ltd.

attorneys if a lawsuit is filed, the Drug Enforcement Administration (DEA) and government auditors who monitor nursing facilities. This chapter provides examples of cases that resulted in actions against APRNs by each of these entities. These examples are from the author's client experience which focuses on nurse practitioners (NPs) or from Board of Nursing websites.

CASES INVOLVING BOARDS OF NURSING

Boards of Nursing have the legal responsibility to investigate APRNs who are reported for incompetence or unprofessional conduct. Reports may come from other nurses, other healthcare professionals, supervisors, patients, or families. If a Board's investigation confirms that an APRN deviated from the standard of care or that an APRN acted unprofessionally, then the Board may discipline the APRN. Discipline may include a "letter of education" which is a letter describing the incident that is placed in the nurse's file but is not accessible to the public. Other types of discipline include a fine, probation, a suspended license, or revocation of a license. The Board also might restrict the nurse's practice, for example, prohibit a nurse midwife from performing deliveries, require continuing education, or require a preceptor to review prescribing and practice. The following examples highlight situations in which NPs were required to defend themselves before Boards of Nursing and the lessons learned.

NP prescribing inconsistent with standard of care

A Board of Nursing charged an NP with incompetence after the NP prescribed Synthroid® for a patient without a diagnosis of hypothyroidism. The NP intended to increase the appetite of the patient, an elderly woman who lived in a nursing home. The NP claimed she discussed this unusual therapeutic approach with her collaborating physician who concurred. However, she did not document this discussion. A nursing home auditor identified the NP's activities and reported her to the Board of Nursing.

Another NP prescribed an extremely large amount of a controlled medication to a man who subsequently sold the pills to a high school student. The student unintentionally overdosed and died. As part of a criminal investigation, the NP was reported to the Board of Nursing for failure to practice according to the standard of care. The NP had not documented an adequate assessment, ongoing monitoring, or a rationale for the large number of pills.

Lesson learned
APRNs are responsible for prescribing within the standard of care which is prescribing a medication for an appropriate indication and at an appropriate dose. Accepted dosage ranges may be found in drug reference books and databases commonly used by APRNs. These include Epocrates® (www.epocrates.com) and Physicians Drug Reference (www.pdr.net) among others. In the first case, there was no clinical indication for Synthroid. If the NP wanted to try an unusual treatment for anorexia, one approach would be to document a resource which provided evidence of effectiveness for her proposed course of treatment. In the second case, if the NP thought it necessary to prescribe large amounts of a controlled medication, the NP should have documented the rationale for that decision.

NP failed to monitor the effect of prescribed medications
An NP prescribed Coumadin® and ordered INR testing every 2 weeks but did not adjust the Coumadin dose in response to results. The patient's INR was at nontherapeutic levels for several months. An auditor for Medicaid reported the NP to the Board of Nursing, and the NP was charged with incompetence.

Lesson learned
NPs are responsible for practicing within the standard of care that includes responding appropriately to laboratory results. In this case, the NP should have increased the dosage of Coumadin in response to test results which showed that the patient was not adequately anticoagulated.

NP prescribed for self or family
An NP prescribed a small amount of anti-anxiety medication for herself. A pharmacist reported her to the Board of Nursing and she is being investigated.

Another NP prescribed a controlled analgesic for her husband who had back pain. A pharmacist reported the NP to the Board of

Nursing and to her employer. The employer fired the NP, and the Board of Nursing investigated.

Lesson learned

APRNs are never authorized to prescribe controlled substances for themselves or relatives. Pharmacists and licensing boards are likely to assume that the APRN is self-medicating. When the pharmacist identifies that the patient and prescriber are related, he/she is obligated to report the irregularity to the prescriber's licensing board. APRNs who prescribe a controlled substance for a patient with the same last name might avoid unnecessary reports by a note on the prescription "patient not related to clinician" or by a conversation with the pharmacist.

NP prescribed outside of legal authority

An NP prescribed a Schedule II medication when NPs in the state were authorized to prescribe only Schedules III–V. The Board of Nursing disciplined the NP.

Another NP who did not have DEA registration prescribed a controlled substance because her physician collaborator agreed to "cover her." A pharmacist reported the NP to the Board of Nursing, who investigated and disciplined the NP.

Lesson learned

Each state's law specifies which of the schedules for controlled substances NPs may prescribe. NPs may not prescribe outside of that authority. Only NPs with DEA registration may prescribe controlled substances. If a patient requires a medication that the APRN is unable to prescribe, alternate procedures could be used such as consultation with a colleague who writes the prescription.

NP altered records to correct prescribing error

An NP was informed by a physician that she had written the wrong dose of an over-the-counter laxative in a consultation letter. The NP replaced the consultation letter with a revised version. The physician noticed that the new version did not match the original, and reported the NP to the Board of Nursing for altering medical records. The Board of Nursing investigated, required the NP to educate herself about the appropriate method for correcting an error in the medical record, and placed a "letter of education" in the NP's file.

Lesson learned

The appropriate way to correct a typewritten record is to add a typed or handwritten addendum. For example, "I wrote in my progress note on May 12, 2010 that I recommended a Milk of Magnesia dose of 1 tablespoon twice a day; however, I told the patient that the dose was 1 teaspoon twice a day. I contacted the patient by telephone and explained the correct dose and confirmed the patient's understanding."

CASES INVOLVING MALPRACTICE ATTORNEYS

If a medical mishap occurs and a patient suffers an injury, the patient may sue the clinician and the clinician's employer for malpractice. For the patient, known as a plaintiff, to mount a successful malpractice case, the patient must prove four elements:

1. that the clinician owed the patient a duty of care
2. that the clinician breached the standard of care
3. that there was an injury
4. that the injury was caused by the breach of the standard of care.

The standard of care is defined in common law (case law) as that degree of care and diligence exercised by a reasonably prudent clinician of similar education and training. Expert witnesses for the plaintiff and defendant(s) will testify as to whether the standard of care was met. The APRN's defense attorney often will argue that one or more of the elements of malpractice were not proven. Examples include the following: it was not proven that there was a duty to the patient; the standard of care was met; there was no injury; or that there was no causal relationship between the breach of the standard of care and the injury. Both the plaintiff's attorney and the defense attorney examine the clinical records related to the patient's care.

The following examples highlight situations in which NPs were required to defend themselves against malpractice claims and the lessons learned.

NP prescribed without legal authority and appropriate monitoring

A hospital-based NP dramatically increased pain medication dosages for a postoperative patient. The patient had a history of medication abuse and was on methadone as well as analgesics. Nurses had asked the NP to increase the analgesics as the patient's pain was not well controlled. Shortly after the NP increased the medication dosages, the patient went into respiratory arrest. The patient was resuscitated but sued the hospital and the NP claiming his cognitive status was not the same after the arrest. The patient's attorneys claimed that the NP's dosages were not within the standard of care, that the NP should have had the patient put on a monitor, and that the NP did not have the legal authority to prescribe the medications she prescribed. The incident occurred in Virginia where an NP may perform functions within the practice of medicine if a physician delegates the authority. The NP stated that she had prescribed under the authority of an anesthesiologist at the hospital. However, the anesthesiologist did not recall authorizing the prescription. At the time of this case, NPs in Virginia did not have the legal authority to prescribe Schedule II medications. The plaintiff won damages of over $1 million.

Lesson learned

An NP must have the legal authority to prescribe. State laws specify if prescriptive authority includes legend drugs (drugs requiring a prescription), controlled substances, or both. State law also regulates which controlled substances may be prescribed and under what circumstances. In the state where this case was filed, NPs may practice medicine if a physician delegates his or her authority. In this case, the NP stated the anesthesiologist at the hospital delegated his authority which he denied.

If a plaintiff's attorney can argue effectively that an NP had no authority to prescribe, then a judge or jury is likely to find that the NP breached the standard of care. In this case, the NP's actions would have been more easily defended had the NP had the delegated authority in writing. The NP's prescribing of Schedule II medications was not authorized by state law. Furthermore, the NP increased the dosages of analgesics to a point where continuous monitoring was indicated but not ordered. The plaintiff's attorney likely argued that this failure was a breach of the standard of care. NPs must meet the clinical standard of care and must have the legal authority to provide any services rendered.

CASES INVOLVING THE DEA

The DEA is the federal agency charged with enforcing the Controlled Substances Act which governs the manufacture, distribution, prescribing, and possession of controlled substances. Pharmacists or other individuals who suspect that an unauthorized health professional is prescribing controlled substances may report the clinician to the DEA. The DEA will investigate, and, if necessary, prosecute the clinician through the U.S. Attorney's Office. The following is a case in which an NP was investigated by the DEA.

A recently graduated NP without DEA registration prescribed a Schedule II medication without realizing that it was controlled. A pharmacist reported her to the DEA. DEA agents arrived at her office and interrogated her. The DEA ultimately decided not to press charges, but her employer was embarrassed by her error and by the DEA visit and fired her.

Lesson learned

APRNs who prescribe controlled substances must have DEA registration and prescribe only those schedules allowed by state law. NPs who do not have DEA registration are responsible for knowing whether a medication they intend to prescribe is controlled. Therefore, APRNs should have an up-to-date list of scheduled drugs and refer to it prior to prescribing. Electronic medication programs such as Epocrates® include information about whether a medication is controlled and update this information regularly.

Controlled substances are listed under Schedules I–V at http:// www.justice.gov/dea/pubs/scheduling.html.

CASES INVOLVING GOVERNMENT AUDITORS

Nursing facilities must comply with Medicare and Medicaid Conditions of Participation. Periodically, Medicare and Medicaid send auditors into nursing facilities to determine whether the federal and state standards for facilities are being met. Auditors review patient records. If an auditor believes that a clinician practicing in the facility has not met the standard of care, the auditor reports the clinician to the appropriate licensing board. The following case highlights a situation in which an auditor reported an NP.

A NP working in a nursing facility gave a verbal order to a nurse to discontinue a medication but did not document it in the record. An auditor for Medicaid reviewed the record and noticed that the orders were not consistent with the care plan. The auditor reported the NP to the Board of Nursing. The Board investigated and charged the NP with incompetence.

Lesson learned
Most facilities have procedures for verbal orders. Generally, the clinician giving the order must cosign the order within 24 hours. In this case, the NP should have written the order to discontinue the medication.

Summary of lessons learned
These cases emphasize that APRNs must have legal authority to prescribe and must meet the standard of care of a reasonably prudent APRN. There are a variety of ways APRNs who are practicing outside of their legal authority or who are not adhering to the standard of care may be identified and reported to regulatory and law enforcement agencies. Therefore, APRNs must be knowledgeable of clinical standards and legal parameters. Clinical standards include:

- Correct dosages
- An accepted indication for each medication prescribed
- Special considerations when prescribing controlled substances for pain
- Monitoring and follow-up of a prescription.

    Legal parameters include:

- Which medications the NP has the legal authority to prescribe under state law
- Which medications are controlled and subject to state and federal regulation
- Limitations on clinician prescribing
- Requirements associated with correcting a prescribing error.

The prescribing practitioner is responsible for ensuring that each prescription conforms to all requirements of the law and regulations, both federal and state. All APRNs have legal parameters for their prescribing.

FEDERAL PRESCRIBING LAWS

Federal prescribing laws focus on controlled substances. A controlled substance is a drug or chemical substance whose possession and use are regulated under the Controlled Substances Act (DEA, 2010a). The DEA has the authority to enforce the Controlled Substances Act. Federal requirements regarding prescriptions address who may prescribe, the purpose of the prescription, the form of the prescription, and how refills may be ordered.

Who may prescribe controlled substances?

Clinicians authorized by state law may prescribe controlled substances if they have registered with the DEA. The DEA's *Practitioner's Manual* (DEA, 2010b) is an important document for APRNs to review as it contains the details of federal requirements of prescribers.

Purpose of a controlled substance prescription

According to the DEA *Practitioner's Manual*, a prescription for a controlled substance, to be valid, must be issued for a legitimate medical purpose by a practitioner acting in the usual course of professional practice. An order purporting to be a prescription issued not in the usual course of professional treatment or in legitimate and authorized research is an invalid prescription according to the Controlled Substances Act. The person who knowingly fills an invalid prescription, as well as the person who writes it, is subject to penalties.

An individual practitioner may not write a prescription for controlled substances with the intention of supplying the practitioner with controlled substances to dispense to patients. According to the DEA *Practitioner's Manual*, a prescription for a controlled substance must be dated and signed on the date when it is written. Federal law prohibits the presigning of prescriptions (Code of Federal Regulations—21 CFR §1306.05, n.d.). If the prescription is not to be dispensed until a date in the future, that should be noted on the prescription as well. The prescription must include the patient's full name and address, and the practitioner's full name, address, and DEA registration number. The prescription must also include:

- drug name
- strength
- dosage form
- quantity prescribed
- directions for use
- number of refills (if any) authorized.

A prescription for a controlled substance must be written in ink or indelible pencil or typewritten and must be manually signed by the practitioner on the date when issued. A practitioner may designate an individual (e.g., a nurse or medical assistant) who may prepare a prescription for the practitioner's signature; however, the practitioner is responsible for the accuracy of the prescription.

Restrictions on amounts prescribed

There is no federal restriction limiting the amount of medication prescribed, although some states do specify limits. An APRN who prescribes extremely large doses or quantities of controlled substances may come to the attention of the DEA or a Board of Nursing and may be investigated and disciplined. The investigators may assume that the APRN is careless or diverting drugs. APRNs who have a legitimate reason for prescribing large amounts should carefully document their rationale in the patient's medical record.

Special rules for schedule II substances

The DEA's *Practitioner's Manual* contains specific rules that pertain only to prescribing Schedule II controlled substances. They require a written prescription that must be signed by the practitioner. In an emergency, a practitioner may call in a prescription for a Schedule II controlled substance. The pharmacist may dispense the prescription provided the quantity prescribed is limited to the amount adequate to treat the patient during the emergency period. The prescribing practitioner must provide a written and signed prescription to the pharmacist within 7 days. The pharmacist must notify the DEA if the prescription is not received.

There is no federal expiration date for a Schedule II prescription; however, states may have time limits. For example, a Schedule II prescription in Washington is valid for 1 year while a similar prescription in Oregon is valid for 2 years. While some states and many insurance companies limit the quantity of controlled substance dispensed to a 30-day supply, there are no specific federal limits to quantities of drugs dispensed via a prescription. The APRN, however, may want to limit the quantity and specify on the prescription that it must last a period of time such as 30 days.

Refilling a prescription for a controlled substance listed in Schedule II is prohibited. There are situations when an APRN may need to prescribe a controlled substance for use a few months in the future. For example, in August, an APRN decides to prescribe the September and October supply of Ritalin® for a student who will be away at college. The legal mechanism is to use the date in August when the prescriptions are written, and indicate "Do not fill until" with the appropriate date in September and October. The DEA's *Practitioner's Manual* says:

An individual practitioner may issue multiple prescriptions authorizing the patient to receive a total of up to a 90-day supply of a Schedule II controlled substance provided certain conditions are met.

- Each separate prescription is issued for a legitimate medical purpose by an individual practitioner acting in the usual course of professional practice.
- The individual practitioner provides written instructions on each prescription (other than the first prescription, if the prescribing practitioner intends for that prescription to be filled immediately) indicating the earliest date on which a pharmacy may fill each prescription.
- The individual practitioner concludes that providing the patient with multiple prescriptions in this manner does not create an undue risk of diversion or abuse.
- The issuance of multiple prescriptions is permissible under applicable state laws.

- The individual practitioner complies fully with all other applicable requirements under the Controlled Substances Act and Code of Federal Regulations, as well as any additional requirements under state law.

The DEA's *Practitioner's Manual* warns that the rules should not be construed as encouraging individual practitioners to issue multiple prescriptions or to see their patients only once every 90 days when prescribing Schedule II controlled substances. Rather, the individual practitioner's decision to issue multiple prescriptions and how often to evaluate patients when doing so should be based on sound clinical judgment and in accordance with established APRN standards.

A prescriber may transmit a Schedule II prescription to the pharmacy by facsimile. The original Schedule II prescription, however, must be presented to the pharmacist for review prior to the actual dispensing of the controlled substance. There are three circumstances in which the facsimile of a Schedule II prescription may serve as the original prescription.

- A practitioner prescribing Schedule II narcotic controlled substances to be compounded for the direct administration to a patient by parenteral, intravenous, intramuscular, subcutaneous or intraspinal infusion may transmit the prescription by facsimile. The pharmacy will consider the facsimile prescription a "written prescription," and no further prescription verification is required. All normal requirements of a legal prescription must be followed.
- Practitioners prescribing Schedule II substances for residents of Long Term Care Facilities may transmit a prescription by facsimile to the dispensing pharmacy. The practitioner's agent may also transmit the prescription to the pharmacy.
- A practitioner prescribing a Schedule II controlled substance for a patient enrolled in a hospice care program certified and/or paid for by Medicare under Title XVIII or a hospice program which is licensed by the state may transmit a prescription to the dispensing pharmacy by facsimile. The practitioner or the practitioner's agent may transmit the prescription to the

pharmacy. The practitioner or agent will note on the prescription that it is for a hospice patient.

Schedule III–V substances

A practitioner may communicate a prescription for controlled substances in Schedules III, IV, and V orally, in writing, or by facsimile to the pharmacist. An oral prescription must be promptly written by the pharmacist containing all information required for a valid prescription, except for the signature of the practitioner. The prescription may be refilled if authorized up to five times within 6 months after the date on which the prescription was issued. After five refills or after 6 months, whichever occurs first, a new prescription is required.

Prescriptions for Schedules III–V controlled substances may be transmitted by facsimile from the practitioner or an employee or agent of the individual practitioner to the dispensing pharmacy. The facsimile is considered to be equivalent to an original prescription.

Delivery of a controlled substance to persons outside the United States

Controlled substances that are dispensed pursuant to a legitimate prescription may not be delivered or shipped to individuals in another country. Any such delivery or shipment is a prohibited export under federal law.

How to avoid problems prescribing controlled substances

Thousands of health professionals prescribe controlled substances and only a very small amount of controlled substances are prescribed for patients without a legitimate need. There are relatively few health professionals who are investigated by state boards and the DEA. An APRN, however, assumes some risks when prescribing controlled substances. First, there is the risk that the patient will divert the drugs. Second, the APRN may become known as a source of controlled drugs in the community. Third, a pharmacist may report the APRN to the licensing board and the DEA if the pharmacist believes the dosages or amounts prescribed are inappropriately high. Even though the dosages or amounts may be correct, APRNs will be expected to provide rationale for their prescribing decisions. Fourth, a patient may decide to sue the APRN, claiming that inappropriate prescribing contributed to the patient's addiction.

While it is impossible to control a patient's behavior, the DEA and Boards of Nursing expect APRNs to be vigilant and refuse prescribing to individuals suspected of selling or diverting drugs. However, the DEA provides no guidance to assist in identifying these individuals.

An important strategy to avoid problems with prescribing scheduled drugs is vigilance about the factors noted by the DEA as indicative of inappropriate prescribing. These include:

- The clinician prescribed inordinately large quantity of controlled substances.
- The clinician issued large numbers of prescriptions for controlled substances.
- No physical examination was documented.
- The clinician warned the patient to fill prescriptions at different pharmacies.
- The clinician issued multiple prescriptions to a patient.
- The clinician prescribed controlled drugs at intervals inconsistent with legitimate medical treatment.
- The clinician used street slang rather than medical terminology for the drugs prescribed.
- There was no logical relationship between the drugs prescribed and treatment of the alleged condition.
- The clinician wrote more than one prescription for same drug at one visit.

Another strategy to avoid problems when prescribing controlled substances is to consider referral to a pain specialist for patients with chronic noncancer pain when one or more of the following situations exist.

- The patient's pain is not well controlled.
- Multiple symptoms require management.
- The patient is unable to care for himself, and caregivers are inconsistent, strained, or burned out.
- The clinician suspects medication abuse.
- The patient has a history of abusing medications.
- There are psychiatric diagnoses or symptoms.

Ask the consultant to evaluate your plan, or ask the consultant to offer a plan for managing the patient's pain. Evaluate the effectiveness of the plan and document any necessary changes.

One attorney (Bolen, 2008) listed mistakes commonly made by clinicians who prescribe controlled substances:

- Failure to respond to patient behaviors
- Poor documentation of referrals
- Failure to justify continued use of pain medication
- Increase in pain medication without rationale
- Use of a benzodiazepine plus opioids without a documented rationale.

Make reasonable efforts to prevent diversion. These include:

- Require periodic urine drug screens of patients taking opioids
- Use face-to-face interviews rather than telephone or e-mail to evaluate patients
- Obtain prior health records and history
- Inquire about prior experience with recreational drugs
- Document all of the precautions noted above.

Follow-up visits should include evaluation of:

- Analgesia (rating of effectiveness on a scale 0–10) compared with prior visit
- Ability to perform activities of daily living such as driving, cooking, walking the dog
- A patient who takes controlled substances and drives may present a risk to self or others. Part of counseling a patient may include advice not to drive. For example, a physician was found liable for failure to warn a patient taking multiple medications not to drive after the patient hit and fatally injured a young boy.
- Adverse effects
- Aberrant drug-related behaviors such as requests for early refills.

Record-keeping requirements

The DEA's *Practitioner's Manual* specifies requirements for record-keeping when prescribing, dispensing, and administering controlled substances. It is necessary to record scheduled drugs if they are dispensed at the practice site. There is no requirement to keep records of controlled substances that are administered. However, practitioners who regularly engage in the dispensing or administering of controlled substances and charge patients a fee for the substances, separately or together with other professional services, must also keep records.

Each practitioner must maintain inventories and records of controlled substances listed as Schedule II, and these must be separate from all other records maintained by the registrant. Likewise, inventories and records of controlled substances in Schedules III, IV, and V must be maintained separate from other records, or in such a form that they are readily retrievable from the ordinary business records of the practitioner. All records related to controlled substances must be maintained and be available for inspection for a minimum of 2 years.

Scheduled drugs that are prescribed for pharmacy dispensing require only the usual chart note (medication, dose, route, timing, amount, and refills, if any) as part of the lawful course of professional practice. Note, however, that state laws may require that clinicians keep records of controlled substances prescribed or copies of prescriptions.

Disposal of controlled substances

A practitioner may dispose of out-of-date, damaged, or otherwise unusable or unwanted controlled substances, including samples, by transferring them to a registrant who is authorized to receive such materials. These registrants are referred to as "reverse distributors." The practitioner should contact the local DEA field office for a list of authorized reverse distributors and use the appropriate process and forms.

Requirements regarding prescription pads

As of October, 1, 2008, federal law requires the use of tamper-resistant prescription pads for Medicaid fee-for-service patients. More than a dozen states have prescription security laws either for all prescriptions or for controlled substances prescriptions. The federally required security features on these pads include:

- Photocopying of a completed or blank prescription is prevented
- No erasure or modification is possible
- No counterfeiting is possible.

In some states, additional security features may be required.

Prescribing off-label

The prescribing of a medication for an indication or dose not specified in the drug manufacturer's insert is referred to as prescribing off-label. There is no law against prescribing off-label. APRNs who prescribe for children typically prescribe off-label as few drugs have been tested in children. However, if an APRN prescribes off-label and the patient is injured and sues, the APRN faces a difficult situation. The presumption regarding standard of care is that drugs are prescribed in accordance with manufacturer's label instructions. Therefore, the APRN will need to rebut the presumption that the off-label medication is not within the standard of care. Consequently, prescribers need to carefully weigh the benefits and risks of prescribing off-label and proceed with caution. Discuss with the patient or parent the rationale for prescribing off-label, obtain their approval, and document the discussion and approval.

STATE LAWS ON PRESCRIBING
Authority to prescribe

NPs and certified nurse-midwives in all states and the District of Columbia may prescribe, order, or furnish medications. However, the legal authority for prescribing is defined differently across the states. Some states, such as Ohio, authorize NPs to prescribe medications specified in a formulary. Others, such as Georgia and Illinois, allow NPs to prescribe if a physician delegates prescriptive authority to the NP. In California, NPs may "furnish" medications under "standardized procedures." Clinical nurse specialists may prescribe in 34 states and the District of Columbia and certified registered nurse anesthetists (CRNAs) in 28 states and the District of Columbia (Kaplan, Brown, & Simonson, 2011; National Council of State Boards of Nursing, 2010).

State laws usually address whether or not a nurse must prescribe under a written agreement with a physician, what must appear on the prescription, which classes of drugs may be prescribed, how to obtain prescriptive authority, and how to maintain prescriptive authority. An example of one state's law regarding NPs is provided in text Box 8.1.

Box 8.1 An example of state law authorizing APRN prescribing

Pennsylvania

A CRNP may prescribe and dispense a drug relevant to the area of practice of the CRNP from the following categories if that authorization is documented in the collaborative agreement (unless the drug is limited or excluded under this or another subsection):

(1) Antihistamines.
(2) Anti-infective agents.
(3) Antineoplastic agents, unclassified therapeutic agents, devices, and pharmaceutical aids if originally prescribed by the collaborating physician and approved by the collaborating physician for ongoing therapy.
(4) Autonomic drugs.
(5) Blood formation, coagulation, and anticoagulation drugs, and thrombolytic and antithrombolytic agents.
(6) Cardiovascular drugs.
(7) Central nervous system agents, except that the following drugs are excluded from this category:
  (i) General anesthetics.
  (ii) Monoamine oxidase inhibitors.
(8) Contraceptives including foams and devices.
(9) Diagnostic agents.
(10) Disinfectants for agents used on objects other than skin.
(11) Electrolytic, caloric, and water balance.
(12) Enzymes.
(13) Antitussive, expectorants, and mucolytic agents.
(14) Gastrointestinal drugs.
(15) Local anesthetics.
(16) Eye, ear, nose, and throat preparations.
(17) Serums, toxoids, and vaccines.
(18) Skin and mucous membrane agents.
(19) Smooth muscle relaxants.
(20) Vitamins.
(21) Hormones and synthetic substitutes.

A CRNP may not prescribe or dispense a drug from the following categories:

(1) Gold compounds.
(2) Heavy metal antagonists.

(3) Radioactive agents.
(4) Oxytocics.

Source: Pa. Regs. §21.284(b)–(c).

Restrictions on CRNP prescribing and dispensing practices are as follows:

(1) A CRNP may write a prescription for a Schedule II controlled substance for up to a 72-hour dose. The CRNP shall notify the collaborating physician as soon as possible but in no event longer than 24 hours.
(2) A CRNP may prescribe a Schedule III or IV controlled substance for up to 30 days. The prescription is not subject to refills unless the collaborating physician authorizes refills for that prescription.

A CRNP may not:

(1) Prescribe or dispense a Schedule I controlled substance as defined in Section 4 of the Controlled Substance, Drug, Device and Cosmetic Act (35 P. S. §780-14).
(2) Prescribe or dispense a drug for a use not approved by the United States Food and Drug Administration without approval of the collaborating physician.
(3) Delegate prescriptive authority specifically assigned to the CRNP by the collaborating physician to another healthcare provider.

A prescription blank shall bear the certification number of the CRNP, name of the CRNP in printed format at the top of the blank, and a space for the entry of the DEA registration number, if appropriate. The collaborating physician shall also be identified as required in §16.91 (relating to identifying information on prescriptions and orders for equipment and service).

The CRNP shall document in the patient's medical record the name, amount, and dose of the drug prescribed, the number of refills, the date of the prescription, and the CRNP's name.

Source: Pa. Regs §21.284 (e)–(h).

There are several resources that provide an overview of state law on prescribing by APRNs or NPs. The resources include: The Pearson Report published each February which can be accessed at http://www.pearsonreport.com/; the annual legislative update published each January in the journal *The Nurse Practitioner*, and a summary in Medscape at http://www.medscape.com/viewarticle/440315. Each APRN should read and understand the law of the state in which the APRN is licensed and practices.

Physician involvement

States vary considerably regarding physician involvement with APRN prescribing. In 13 states and the District of Columbia, APRNs are fully independent with no physician involvement in prescribing (Pearson, 2011). In other states, physicians must sign a document authorizing an APRN to prescribe. These documents may be called written collaborative agreements, delegating documents, protocols, or standardized procedures. Box 8.2 is an example of Kansas state law regarding physician participation with NPs who prescribe.

Form of prescription

State laws vary regarding what the prescription must contain. In general, state laws require that a prescription include the patient's name, date, medication, dose, route, frequency, and name, credential, address, and telephone number of the prescribing NP. Some states require the name, address, and telephone number of the collaborating physician.

Box 8.2 Kansas State law on physician collaboration for prescribing

An advanced registered nurse practitioner may prescribe drugs pursuant to a written protocol as authorized by a responsible physician. Each written protocol shall contain a precise and detailed medical plan of care for each classification of disease or injury for which the advanced registered nurse practitioner is authorized to prescribe and shall specify all drugs which may be prescribed by the advanced registered nurse practitioner. Any written prescription order shall include the name, address, and telephone number of the responsible physician. The advanced registered nurse practitioner may not dispense drugs, but may request, receive, and sign for professional samples and may distribute professional samples to patients pursuant to a written protocol as authorized by a responsible physician (Kansas State Statutes, 2000).

Prescribing for self or family members

APRNs should avoid prescribing for family members, unless the family member is enrolled at a practice where the APRN regularly diagnoses and treats patients.

While there may be no law specifically prohibiting an APRN from prescribing legend drugs, such as antibiotics, for family members, there are legal reasons for declining to do so. APRNs are particularly vulnerable in states that require a collaborative agreement with a physician. Collaborative agreements are specific to a practice setting; therefore, the family member must be enrolled as a patient at the APRN's practice setting in order to prescribe. In states where no collaborative agreement is required, an NP who prescribes for a family member is on somewhat firmer ground.

Prescribing legend drugs for one's self is also inadvisable. The APRN should consider that this is not likely to be covered under a collaborative agreement. Furthermore, self-prescribing does not provide the APRN as a patient with the best health care possible. The Arkansas Board of Nursing provides practice guidance on this matter in a position statement (Box 8.3).

Prescribing controlled substances for family members or oneself carries even greater risks. Pharmacy laws make it illegal in many states to prescribe controlled substances for family members or self. Ohio law, for example, provides guidance on this issue (Box 8.4).

Even if it is not expressly illegal under many state laws to prescribe a controlled substance for a family member, it is always inadvisable. The pharmacist may suspect that the prescriber, rather than the family member, is using the drug personally and make a report to the licensing board. The APRN may then be in the position of having to prove that he or she is not self-administering controlled substances. Furthermore, DEA registration is specific to a practice setting. An APRN who prescribes a controlled substance for a family member who is not a patient in the practice may be violating two laws.

How long are prescriptions valid?

State laws vary regarding the length of time that prescriptions are valid. The typical prescription is valid for 1 year.

Box 8.3 Arkansas Board of Nursing position statement on prescribing for self and family members

Prescribing controlled substances and other legend drugs for self and family raises many ethical questions. Prescribing for self and family members has inherent risks related to lack of objectivity. Effort should be made to discuss the condition with the collaborating physician. In addition, the *Arkansas State Board of Nursing Rules and Regulations* (Chapter Four. Section VIII.D.5) outlines the documentation requirements for prescribing.

The Arkansas State Board of Nursing has determined that the advanced practice nurse (APN) with prescriptive authority may prescribe for self and family under the following circumstances:

1. There shall be a medical record on the patient/client to document the prescription of the medication.
2. The prescription must be within the prescriber's scope of practice.
3. The prescription shall be documented on the medical record in accordance with *Arkansas State Board of Nursing Rules and Regulations*.

The APN shall note prescriptions on the client's medical record and include the following information:

a. Medication and strength
b. Dose
c. Amount prescribed
d. Directions for use
e. Number of refills; and
f. Initials or signature of APN.

Source: Arkansas State Board of Nursing, 1999.

Formularies

Some state laws list the medications APRNs may prescribe; other state laws have more general language. For example, Ohio has a formulary which specifies drugs that may be initiated by the APRN and drugs that may be prescribed only after the collaborating physician has examined the patient or consulted with the APRN.

**Box 8.4 Ohio State Board of Pharmacy standards for
prescribing controlled substances for self or family members**

Accepted and prevailing standards of care presuppose a professional
relationship between a patient and practitioner when the practitioner is
utilizing controlled substances. By definition, a practitioner may never
have such a relationship with himself or herself. Thus, a practitioner
may not self-prescribe or self-administer controlled substances. . . .
Accepted and prevailing standards of care require that a practitioner
maintain detached professional judgment when utilizing controlled substances in the treatment of family members. A practitioner shall utilize
controlled substances when treating a family member only in an emergency situation which shall be documented in the patient's record. For
the purposes of this rule, "family member" means a spouse, parent,
child, sibling, or other individual in relation to whom a practitioner's
personal or emotional involvement may render the practitioner unable
to exercise detached professional judgment in reaching diagnostic or
therapeutic decisions.

Source: Ohio State Board of Pharmacy, 1998.

Standard of care regarding prescribing

Few health professions have rules or position statements that
delineate policies on prescribing. Only one major nursing organization, the American Nurses Association (ANA), has published a
standard of care regarding prescribing. Standard 5D of ANA's
(2010) *Nursing: Scope and Standards of Practice* establishes a standard
and a set of competencies for APRN prescriptive authority. At the
time of this writing, no federal agency has established standards
of care regarding prescribing. Some specialty organizations,
however, have standards of care regarding prescribing and administering medications. For example, the American Pain Society
(2009) has standards for prescribing controlled substances for
chronic noncancer pain. The Oncology Nursing Society and
American Society of Clinical Oncology (2009) have standards
regarding administration of chemotherapy.

Policies may exist at the state or institutional level. One policy
from the Tennessee Board of Medical Examiners titled *Prerequisites*

Box 8.5 Tennessee State Board of Medical Examiners prerequisites to prescribing or dispensing drugs in person, electronically, or over the Internet

(1) Except as provided in paragraph (2), it shall be a prima facie violation of T.C.A. 63-6-214 (b) (1), (4), and (12) for a physician to prescribe or dispense any drug to any individual, whether in person or by electronic means, or over the Internet or over telephone lines, unless the physician has first done and appropriately documented, for the person to whom a prescription is to be issued or drugs dispensed, all of the following:

(a) Performed an appropriate history and physical examination;
(b) Made a diagnosis based upon the examinations and all diagnostic and laboratory tests consistent with good medical care;
(c) Formulated a therapeutic plan, and discussed it, along with the basis for it and the risks and benefits of various treatments options, a part of which might be the prescription or dispensing drug, with the patient; and
(d) Insured availability of the physician or coverage for the patient for appropriate follow-up care.

(2) A physician may prescribe or dispense drugs for a person not in compliance with subparagraph (a) in circumstances including, but not limited to, the following:

(a) In admission orders for a newly hospitalized patient;
(b) For a patient of another physician for whom the prescriber is taking calls;
(c) For continuation medications on a short-term basis for a new patient prior to the patient's first appointment; and
(d) For established patients who, based on sound medical practices, the physician feels does not require a new physical examination before issuing new prescriptions.

Source: Tennessee Board of Medical Examiners, 2000.

---

to Prescribing or Dispensing Drugs—in Person, Electronically or Over the Internet is equally applicable to APRNs (Box 8.5).

Nurses Service Organization (NSO), a company which insures NPs against professional liability, studied the reasons why NPs were sued from 1998–2008 (CNA Healthpro, 2010). NSO's findings related to prescribing are provided in Table 8.1. Claims related to

Table 8.1 Selected categories of claims related to medication

Allegation	% of closed claims with indemnity payment	Average paid indemnity
Wrong medication	35.9	$174,561
Wrong dose	23.1	$84,085
Failure to properly discontinue medication	12.8	$276,000

Source: CNA Healthpro, 2010.

medication were primarily linked to selecting the wrong medication, selecting the wrong dose, and failing to properly discontinue a medication. Based on these findings, it would seem reasonable to formulate a standard of care for prescribing which includes the following.

- Discontinue medications which are no longer necessary or which cause dangerous side effects.
- Before prescribing, check for incompatibilities with current medications and contraindications based on comorbidities.
- After writing a prescription or drug order, check that you have written for the correct medication, in the correct dose, by the correct route, in the correct timing.
- Check that writing or printing is legible or, preferably, use electronic prescribing technology.

Additional general principles for safe prescribing are as follows (Buppert, 2010):

- With every prescription, go through a SCRIPT analysis:
  - Side effects—*Do I need to alert the patient about what to watch for?*
  - Contraindications—*Do any listed contraindications pertain to this patient? If so, should I prescribe something else?*
  - Right medication, dose, frequency, and route—*Have I checked all of these against a reference?*
  - Interactions—*Might any of the patient's other medications interact with this one? If so, should I prescribe something else?*

- ○ Precautions—*Do any listed precautions pertain to this patient? If so, should I prescribe something else?*
- ○ Transmittal—Is my writing legible to others?
- Write no prescription without an evaluation and documentation in the patient's chart.
- Refer to a pain specialist when appropriate.
- Documentation
  - ○ Keep the refill record in a central place in the chart, rather than documenting refills only in the note for the daily visit.
  - ○ Record prescriptions transmitted to pharmacies while away from the office.
  - ○ Self-audit your own documentation with a critical eye. For example, are all of the patient's medications necessary? One way to avoid risk is to avoid prescribing, unless absolutely necessary. Has the patient received refills of controlled substances only at the appropriate and expected times?
- Counsel patients for whom you have prescribed controlled substances that they should not drive, and document the advice.

CONCLUSION

Knowledge of prescribing laws and attention to standards of care are essential to prevent errors. Once a year, review your state's Board of Nursing website which can be accessed through https://www.ncsbn.org/515.htm. Also review the DEA website at http://www.deadiversion.usdoj.gov/drugreg/index.html. It is imperative that APRNs are knowledgeable about any changes in the rules and policies on prescribing. If prescribing controlled substances, conduct an annual Internet search for new standards set by professional associations or state boards. Attend continuing education programs on prescribing or complete self-study modules online to obtain current information on medication and prescribing practices.

Information provided in this chapter offers guidance to decrease legal risks and avoid difficult situations. Damage caused when prescribing, especially from ill-chosen medications, may be impossible to undo. A patient's legal remedy—monetary damages—never makes the patient whole. Furthermore, the effect on an APRN of a report to a Board of Nursing can be emotionally exhausting and professionally catastrophic. Errors can occur even when providing high-quality care. Prevention of errors is well worth the effort. Attention to professional standards as well as state and federal laws will significantly increase APRN confidence. The prescribing role is an essential component of practice and medications may significantly enhance a patient's quality of life. Despite the challenges, experience and careful attention can create a competent APRN prescriber.

REFERENCES

American Nurses Association. (2010). *Nursing: Scope and standards of practice*. Silver Spring, MD: American Nurses Association.

American Pain Society. (2009). Clinical guidelines for the use of chronic opioid therapy in chronic noncancer pain. Retrieved from http://www.ampainsoc.org/pub/cp_guidelines.htm

American Society of Clinical Oncology. (2009). American society of clinical oncology/oncology nursing society chemotherapy administration safety standards. Retrieved from http://www.asco.org/ASCOv2/Department%20Content/Cancer%20Policy%20and%20Clinical%20Affairs/Downloads/Final%20Standards%20Table.pdf

Arkansas State Board of Nursing. (1999). Chapter four. Section VIII.D.3-5 and Arkansas State Board of Nursing Position Statement 99-3. Retrieved from www.arsbn.arkansas.gov/lawsRules/Documents/99_3.pdf

Bolen, J. (2008). Presentation to the American Academy of Pain Management annual conference.

Buppert, C. (2010). *Prescribing: Preventing legal pitfalls for nurse practitioners*. Bethesda, MD: Law Office of Carolyn Buppert.

CNA Healthpro. (2010). Understanding nurse practitioner liability: CNA Healthpro nurse practitioner claims analysis 1998–2008, risk management strategies and highlights of the 2009 NSO Survey. Retrieved from http://www.nso.com/pdfs/db/Nurse_Practitioner_Claim_Study_02-12-10.pdf?fileName=Nurse_Practitioner_Claim_Study_02-12-10.pdf&folder=pdfs/db&isLiveStr=Y

Code of the Federal Register. (n.d.). §1306.05 Manner of issuance of prescriptions. Retrieved from http://edocket.access.gpo.gov/cfr_2010/aprqtr/pdf/21cfr1306.05.pdf

Drug Enforcement Administration. (2010a). Title 21 United States code (USC) controlled substances act. Retrieved from http://www.deadiversion.usdoj.gov/21cfr/21usc/index.html

Drug Enforcement Administration. (2010b). Practitioner's manual. Retrieved from http://www.deadiversion.usdoj.gov/pubs/manuals/pract/index.html

Kansas Statutes Annotated. (2000). Advanced registered nurse practitioner; standards and requirements for obtaining certificate of qualification; rules and regulations; categories, education, qualifications and role; limitations and restrictions; prescription of drugs authorized §65-1130(d). Retrieved from http://www.ksbn.org/npa/npa.pdf

Kaplan, L., Brown, M. A., & Simonson, D. C. (2011). CRNA prescribing practices: The Washington state experience. *AANA Journal, 79*(1), 24–29.

National Council of State Boards of Nursing. (2010). Member board profiles. https://www.ncsbn.org/2010_Regulation_of_Advanced_Practice_Nursing.pdf

Ohio State Board of Pharmacy. (1998). Rule 4731-11-08 utilizing controlled substances for self and family member. Retrieved from http://pharmacy.ohio.gov/csdiet-001001.htm

Pearson, L. J. (2011). The Pearson report. Retrieved from http://www.pearsonreport.com

Tennessee State Board of Medical Examiners. (2000). Prerequisites to prescribing or dispensing drugs in person, electronically or over the internet. Retrieved from http://health.state.tn.us/Downloads/g3010259.pdf

The Role of Cultural Competence in Prescribing Medications

9

Mary Sobralske, Louise Kaplan, and Marie Annette Brown

This chapter explores cultural influences in pharmacotherapy including biological variation, race, ethnicity, primary language, literacy, socio-economics, disabilities, and religious beliefs. Factors related to ethno-pharmacology can also affect selection of particular medications. Understanding patients' and families' culture and health beliefs contributes to the development of the knowledge and attitudes necessary for prescribing in a culturally appropriate manner.

The cultural and linguistic diversity of the United States is rapidly increasing. Consequently, it is imperative for advanced practice registered nurses (APRNs) to understand the effects of racial and biological variation and the cultural and ethnic influences on health and health care. Cultural competence results in an ability to understand, communicate with, and effectively interact with diverse populations. Providing culturally competent care is especially important when developing treatment plans and determining appropriate medications. The capacity to explain medications to patients and their caregivers in a culturally sensitive manner is essential (Teal & Street, 2009).

The Advanced Practice Registered Nurse as a Prescriber, First Edition. Marie Annette Brown, Louise Kaplan.
© 2012 John Wiley & Sons, Ltd. Published 2012 by John Wiley & Sons, Ltd.

Culture, health, and illness are closely linked. Culture is defined as the values, beliefs, rules of behavior, and lifestyle practices of a particular group of people. Cultural values are learned and shared. Cultural beliefs guide thinking, decision making, and actions (Leininger & McFarland, 2006). The patient's worldview and beliefs about health and illness, including use of medications, are also affected by age, concept of time, and ways of communicating. The cultural diversity of populations extends beyond racial and ethnic minorities and people with limited English proficiency. Examples of diverse groups are people who have limited literacy or disabilities, live in poverty, or have varying sexual orientations and religious beliefs. The purpose of this chapter is to discuss the role of cultural competence in prescribing medications.

RACE, ETHNICITY, AND BIOLOGICAL VARIATION
Health disparities

The American Heart Association, in conjunction with several government agencies, published a report on the epidemiology of various health problems and risk factors which highlights racial and ethnic disparities. Hypertension is prevalent among 23% of whites, 21.5% of Hispanics or Latinos, 32.3% of blacks or African Americans, 19.4% of Asians, and 21.8% of American Indians or Alaska Natives. The prevalence of hypertension among African American women is highest of any comparison group at 44%. Cardiovascular disease (CVD) includes hypertension, heart disease, stroke, peripheral artery disease, and diseases of the veins. African American women have a 47.3% prevalence of CVD compared to the prevalence rate of 36.2% for men and women of all races (Roger et al., 2011).

Diabetes is another condition for which there is a great deal of disparity among racial and ethnic groups. White males and females have a prevalence rate for diabetes of 6.8% and 6.5%, respectively, compared to 14.3% and 14.7% for black males and females, and 11% and 12.7% for Mexican American males and females. The prevalence of low-density lipoprotein (LDL) cholesterol ≥130 was highest among Mexican American men at 41.9% compared to the lowest prevalence among black women at 27.7% (Roger et al., 2011).

Conceptualizations of race and ethnicity

Race in the United States has been categorized by placing people into groups based on skin color, eye color, or hair and is often used when conducting health research. Definitions of race also include geographical or country of origin, such as African American. Based on these definitions, racial categories can sometimes be vague and confusing (O'Loughlin, Dugas, Maximova, & Kishchuk, 2006) (Box 9.1).

Because accumulated data in health sciences research reports on racial differences, this discussion of cultural competence will include the concept of race as a consideration in APRN prescribing. Eventually, however, evidence may not rely on the artificially constructed concept of race. Instead, cultural and biological variations will be articulated in a more precise way. New directions in genetics may replace our current understanding of biological variances attributed to race. For example, Franciosa, Ferdinand, and Yancy (2010b) emphasize that in future research "the interface of race/ethnicity and genetics must be managed carefully and where appropriate physiologic markers of disease should be supplanted for race. But race is not a proxy for genetics, and genetic signals are not sufficient to provoke disease and must occur in the setting of certain environmental and clinical factors that promote disease expression" (p. 1).

Box 9.1 The concept of race in transition

Current perspectives question the concept of race. In 2000, the Human Genome Project declared that there was no genetic basis for race (Hamilton, 2008). In fact, 99.9% of all humans share the same genes. Only 0.1% genetic variation accounts for differences among humans. The American Anthropological Association (AAA) (2011) project "*RACE Are We So Different?* looks at race in the United States through the eyes of history, science, and lived experience. The program explains how human variation differs from race, when and why the idea of race was invented, and how race and racism affects everyday life. The program conveys three overall messages: (1) Race is a recent human invention; (2) Race is about culture, not biology; (3) Race and racism are embedded in institutions and everyday life" (http://www.aaanet.org/resources/A-Public-Education-Program.cfm).

In the past, race was most associated with biology while ethnicity was commonly associated with culture. The two concepts, however, are not clearly distinct. The American Anthropological Association [AAA] defines ethnicity as the identification with population groups characterized by common ancestry, language, and custom. However, "because of common origins and intermarriage, ethnic groups often share physical characteristics which also then become a part of their identification by themselves and by others" (AAA, 1997). In addition, populations with similar physical appearance may have a different ethnic identity, and populations with different physical appearances may have a common ethnic identity.

Ethnicity is the perception of oneself and a sense of belonging to a particular group, belonging to more than one group, or a feeling of not belonging to any group. Ethnicity is integral to ethnic pride, identity, affiliation, and loyalty. Ethnicity differs from race and includes more than biological identification. It is the degree of commitment and involvement in important and meaningful cultural customs and rituals. For example, many Filipinos consider it virtuous to accept pain and suffering, and medication may not be requested when it could provide pain relief (Galanti, 2004).

Ethnopharmacology and biological variation

Biological variation in health and illness may be influenced by race, ethnicity, and environmental factors. As a result, some health problems are more common in certain racial and ethnic groups. Conditions such as lactose intolerance and thalassemia, which are found in many Asian, Middle-Eastern, and Latino populations, can affect how individuals absorb and respond to drugs (DeBaun & Vichinsky, 2007; Enattah et al., 2002; Giardina & Forget, 2008). Compared to Caucasians, African Americans are more likely to be salt-sensitive and may benefit from medications that affect serum sodium levels in a positive manner when treating hypertension and kidney disease (Norris, Tareen, Martins, & Vaziri, 2008).

Although genetically all humans are very much alike, research on drug responses has demonstrated that pharmacodynamics and pharmacokinetics can differ across ethnic groups and races. Ethnopharmacology focuses on the effect race and ethnicity has on the responses to medication, drug absorption, metabolism, distribution, and excretion (Muñoz & Hilgenberg, 2005).

Consideration of the patient's race, ethnicity, and biology are components of prescribing decisions. There is evidence that certain racial groups may suffer more adverse effects with particular medications or respond better to some classes of drugs than others (Douglas, 2003; Glazer et al., 1994).

The effect of race and ethnicity on psychotropic and antihypertensive drugs has been the most studied of all drug classes. It is important to note that disparities exist in the utilization of psychotropic drugs among different groups. For example, between 1996 and 2005, the overall rate of antidepressant use doubled in the United States from 5.8% to 10.1%. The rate of use for African Americans in 2005 was only 4.5%, and the rate for Hispanics was only 5.2% (Olfsun & Marcus, 2009).

Knowledge of differences in how racial and ethnic groups manage medications can assist the APRN when making decisions about drug therapy. A study by Turner, Hollenbeak, Weiner, Ten Have, and Roberts (2009) examined barriers to and the effect of adherence to antihypertensive blood pressure medication among racially diverse elderly patients. Compared to other study participants, elderly black patients who reported missing medications within the past 3 months of the study had significantly poorer blood pressure control. Selection of a medication with a simple drug regimen was identified as one consideration in selecting the appropriate medication.

The influence of health beliefs among African American clinic patients to the incidence and control of hypertension also provides important guidance for prescribers. In one study of African Americans with hypertension, 38% believed that they would be cured, 38% did not expect to take antihypertensive medication for life, and 23% thought that antihypertensive medications needed to be taken only when experiencing symptoms (Ogedegbe, Mancuso, & Allegrante, 2004). In the Consensus Statement on Management of Hypertension in Blacks, Flack et al. (2010) highlight data from several studies about nonphysiologic factors linked to poor blood pressure control. Even though blacks perceived this health problem as more significant compared to non-blacks, they experienced greater stress, concern about hypertension, and adverse medication effects, than their counterparts. They also tended to be older and have a recent (past 5 years) diagnosis of hypertension. Difficulty reading, adequately following the medication regimens, and self-reported nonadherence also contributed to the complexity of the situation. This evidence offers further insight to APRNs who are considering multiple factors in the selection of pharmacotherapeutics.

Chaudhry, Neelam, Duddu, and Husain (2008) conducted a review of the literature regarding the relationship between ethnicity and psychopharmacology. Examples of data suggesting a link between ethnicity and clinical response to psychotropic drugs included the following.

- Asian and Hispanic patients required lower doses of antipsychotics to obtain treatment effects similar to those of other ethnic groups.
- Asian patients who received a significantly lower dose of clozapine had blood concentration levels comparable to a Caucasian group.
- Black patients had a therapeutic response to lower doses of tricyclic antidepressants than Caucasian patients.
- Hispanics and Asians developed movement disorders more often than Caucasians despite taking lower doses of chlorpromazine.

Many retrospective studies document the effect of atypical antipsychotic drugs on metabolic risk among patients with schizophrenia; however, few prospective studies have been conducted. One prospective study compared the response of white, black, and Hispanic patients taking aripiprazole (Abilify®) or olanzapine (Zyprexa®). Greater metabolic improvement occurred in patients taking aripiprazole than those on olanzapine. White patients had a more consistent metabolic improvement than the black and Hispanic patients (Meyer, Rosenblatt, Kim, Baker, & Whitehead, 2009). Consideration of multiple facets in the selection of a particular medication is essential with careful monitoring of metabolic risk.

When treating hypertension in African Americans, some drugs may be better suited than others. The article "Management of High Blood Pressure in Blacks: An Update of the International Society on Hypertension in Blacks Consensus Statement" (Flack et al. 2010) notes:

> If blood pressure is 10mm Hg above target levels, monotherapy with a diuretic or calcium channel blocker is preferred. When blood pressure is 15/10mm Hg above target, 2-drug therapy is recommended, with either a calcium channel blocker plus a renin-angiotensin system blocker or, alternatively, in edematous and/or volume-overload states, with a thiazide diuretic plus a renin-angiotensin system blocker. Effective multi-drug therapeutic combinations through 4 drugs are described. Comprehensive lifestyle modifications should be initiated in blacks when blood pressure is ≥ 115/75mm Hg. The updated . . . consensus statement on hypertension management in blacks lowers the minimum target blood pressure level for the lowest-risk blacks, emphasizes effective multidrug regimens, and de-emphasizes monotherapy. (p. 780)

There are other recommendations for specific medications when treating African Americans. For example, isosorbide-hydralyzine (BiDil®) remains the most effective drug for heart failure in African Americans (Franciosa, Ferdinand, & Yancy, 2010a). ACE inhibitors have been found to be less effective than the diuretic chlorthalidone in preventing stroke in African Americans (Furberg et al., 2002).

A study in the United Kingdom of different drug treatments for hypertension revealed some differences among Caucasians, people of African origin, and people of South Asian origin. People of African origin were significantly less responsive to atenolol (Tenormin®) monotherapy compared to Caucasians. However, when a diuretic was added, blood pressure was lowered to a similar extent among the three groups. Response to monotherapy with amlodipine (Norvasc®) did not differ among the three groups. When perindopril (Aceon®) was added to amlodipine, patients of African origin had a lesser response and patients of South-Asian origin a greater response than Caucasian patients (Gupta et al., 2010).

Statins can lower plasma LDL-cholesterol, reduce oxidative stress of body tissue, offer antioxidant effects, reduce inflammation, and stabilize atherosclerotic plaque (Carey, 2010). They are most commonly prescribed to reduce CVD risk. Treatment responses vary across races. Genetic differences may modify both statin efficacy and susceptibility to statin-induced adverse drug reactions (Mangravite, Wilke, Zhang, & Krauss, 2008).

Two genes have been associated with varying responses to warfarin (Coumadin®) dosing for anticoagulation therapy. Dosage requirements differ across race and ethnicity. Asians and Hispanics may require a smaller dose than Caucasians, and African Americans may require more than the standard dose (Johnson, 2008).

PERCEIVED DISCRIMINATION

The history of the United States includes an unfortunate series of events that have created distrust of the healthcare system among African Americans and other racial and ethnic groups. Experiments were conducted on African American slaves, the graves of blacks were plundered to provide bodies to medical schools, and the Tuskegee syphilis experiment was conducted during which patients had treatment withheld without their consent (Gamble, 1997).

Native Americans have also experienced past injustices that cause distrust. The Havasupai Indian tribe in Arizona sued an Arizona State University researcher who collected blood samples to study the high rate of diabetes among the tribal members and subsequently used the samples to conduct experiments regarding mental illness, inbreeding, and population migration. The tribe sued on the basis that members gave permission only to study diabetes which the researcher disputed. The university settled with the tribe in 2010 and paid $700,000 to 41 tribal members, returned the blood samples, and provided other forms of assistance to the tribe (Harmon, 2010).

A recent study explored the experience of African American women with health professionals when they received care. The study revealed that provider behaviors perceived as racially discriminatory included avoidance of touching the patient, assumptions about the patient's financial status, and perceived apathy in making a diagnosis. Study participants expressed mistrust of white providers, expecting to be treated unfairly, a negative emotional reaction to racial discrimination in clinical encounters, and choosing not to return for an appointment if discrimination was perceived (Greer, 2010). Cross-cultural education can increase the sensitivity of APRNs to issues of race, ethnicity, and culture. Using effective communication can also avoid patients perceiving APRNs as discriminatory.

IMMIGRATION, ACCULTURATION, AND ASSIMILATION

Health beliefs are shaped by cultural history and socialization. Socialization occurs as a person learns to live, work, and become an accepted member of a society. People learn what is important and acceptable within a society, including the perception of when medications are needed or desired and how to go about seeking them.

Immigration

Many immigrants to the United States have indigenous health beliefs and social expectations. Some immigrants may be quite surprised to have an APRN of the opposite gender examining and treating them. Consider if a man is from a culture where men are in a position of authority and may resent a female APRN prescribing treatment. Also consider if a female immigrant may be too modest or embarrassed to accept the care of a male APRN.

Some immigrants to the United States may bring a supply of medications and continue to use them without consulting a healthcare provider. Immigrants may have continued access to medication from their countries of origin where they can purchase them directly from pharmacies without a prescription. Many prescription drugs in the United States can be purchased over the counter in Mexico where pharmacists commonly prescribe drugs. These include drugs such as amoxicillin, Premarin®, and Retin A®. Immigrants may not be aware that these medications are prescription drugs in the United States and may also be surprised at the cost when they acquire prescription medications at a U.S. pharmacy.

The level of acculturation can affect a patient's expectation about how a health problem should be treated. As a result of acculturation, a person adopts some traits of the mainstream culture. This can occur slowly over time or quite quickly depending on the circumstances such as rural versus urban living. The American healthcare system with its rules and cultural assumptions can be very confusing to many immigrants (Galanti, 2008). It is particularly confusing to immigrants who do not speak English. As an example, an Asian patient who is less acculturated may expect a prescription for a preparation to be obtained from an herbal pharmacist. A more acculturated patient may expect a prescription for a manufactured antibiotic tablet dispensed at a pharmacy (Galanti, 2008).

Assimilation

Assimilation is a blending of cultural heritage into the social, political, and economic fabric of the mainstream society. Assimilation involves developing a new cultural identity and the realization that one may never return to the society of origin (Clark & Hofsess, 1998). The degree of assimilation influences expectations for treatment and the ability to understand the necessity of prescriptions.

Some Latino immigrants may suffer from *empacho*, a gastrointestinal illness that is perceived to be a stomach or intestinal blockage (Neff, 1999). A commonly held belief in traditional societies is that *empacho* must be treated because it will progress and may even lead to death (Ortiz, Shields, Clauson, & Clay, 2007). A less assimilated patient from Guatemala, Mexico, and Puerto Rico who immigrated to the United States recently may rely on remedies such as *azarcón* and *greta* for empacho. The APRN needs to be aware that *azarcón* and *greta* both contain lead and be alert to the need to evaluate lead levels in the user of these remedies.

Another example of the possible effect of assimilation on prescribing is a 66-year-old man born in the mountains of Laos who chooses not to accept an antibiotic for a prostate infection. He may attribute his illness to soul loss and desire spiritual healing which involves retrieving the lost soul from another plane of existence (Culture Care Connection, 2010).

RELIGIOUS BELIEFS AND MEDICATION

Religion is an organized system of beliefs or symbols concerning order and the meaning of existence (Andrews, 2007). Religious beliefs may dictate ideas, thinking, and behaviors that can influence health. Some beliefs hold that religion and health are inseparable. In certain instances, religious beliefs can affect the acceptance of common primary care treatments and prescription medications. For example, some patients may feel more comfortable with spiritual healing practices such as prayer than prescription medications.

Members of the Church of Christ, Scientist ordinarily do not use any medications (Spector, 2009), and immunizations are only acceptable when required by law (Andrews & Boyle, 2008). Jehovah's Witnesses are forbidden to receive blood and blood products such as clotting factor for hemophilia-related hemarthrosis. The Congregation of Universal Wisdom is opposed to receiving immunizations. Patients who are part of a Hutterite community, a German-dialect speaking Christian ethno-religious group, may be required to defer decisions about health care to a church elder (Fahrenwald, Boysen, Fischer, & Maurer, 2001). When insulin was extracted from pig pancreas, it was considered taboo to use for Jews who keep kosher, dietary rules that prohibit pork. Contraceptive medications and devices are prohibited by certain religions such as the Roman Catholic faith. However, religious affiliation itself may or may not predict a patient's approach to health and healthcare decisions. Individuals of all faiths vary in how they interpret and accept religious tenets. Genuine concern and respect coupled with interest in "knowing the patient" provide the foundation for APRN prescribing.

APRNs may be aware of religious and spiritual objects worn or used to "ward off" illness and protect the individual's health. Objects used to protect health include amulets, talismans, bangles, and ribbons. Substances used to protect health include foods such as cloves of garlic, onion, and thousand-year-old eggs (Spector, 2009). Support for concurrent use of these objects with prescription medications conveys cultural acceptance.

FAMILIES AND PRESCRIBING

It is important to understand the cultural aspects of family dynamics that may influence the implementation of medication regimens. Inclusion of the family member who controls healthcare decision-making may be necessary when prescribing medications. In some cultures, the man is seen as the authority figure outside the home, and the woman is in charge of the household and health care of the children (Galanti, 2008). In other cultures, the grandmother may have the power and authority (Kataoka-Yahiro, Ceria, & Caulfield, 2004). In this situation, the grandmother must agree with the use of a prescribed medication, or the APRN may find a prescription remains unfilled.

Conflicts about medications may occur within families. A husband may disapprove of his wife's desire to use contraception.

If he is present during clinical encounters, approaches to this situation may require the APRN to assist the patient with her negotiation skills or create an opportunity to work with the woman alone. Family members may disagree with each other or an older adult's decision to refuse drug treatment for a terminal illness. An infant's parents or grandparents may believe their child should receive a prescription for antibiotics when the infant has a viral upper respiratory infection. Negotiating with families about antibiotic use requires thoughtful approaches. These are discussed further in Chapter 5 on difficult clinical situations. Childhood immunizations can be a contentious issue in families. Parents may not agree with each other about whether their children will receive them. Depending on cultural beliefs and values, these family disagreements may be confusing for a clinician and require expertise in facilitating family decision making.

COMMUNICATION AND PRESCRIBING

Safe, rational, and appropriate prescribing requires clear communication and attention to both verbal and nonverbal communications. Because communication patterns can vary across cultures, APRNs will need to individualize their approaches. For example, eye contact may be seen as desirable and expected in some cultures and taboo in others, such as in some Native American tribes. Asking the patient "what do you think is wrong and what will make you better?" is an anthropological approach that provides patients the opportunity to disclose their "explanatory model" (Kleinman, 1980). This is the patient's explanation for what is happening and why symptoms are experienced based on cultural and religious beliefs. This may deepen the APRN's cultural understanding of why patients resist, accept, or request medications.

Literacy and limited English proficiency

The National Standards on Culturally and Linguistically Appropriate Services (The Office of Minority Health, 2010) include providing interpreters for patients with limited English proficiency (LEP) (see Box 9.2). When APRNs are not bilingual in healthcare terminology, an interpreter needs to provide the critical link to insure safe and effective treatment decisions. Interpreters can enhance communication and quality of care and are legally required

Box 9.2 National Standards on Culturally and Linguistically Appropriate Services (CLAS)

The CLAS standards are primarily directed at healthcare organizations; however, individual providers are also encouraged to use the standards to make their practices more culturally and linguistically accessible. The principles and activities of culturally and linguistically appropriate services should be integrated throughout an organization and undertaken in partnership with the communities being served.

The 14 standards are organized by themes: Culturally Competent Care (Standards 1–3), Language Access Services (Standards 4–7), and Organizational Supports for Cultural Competence (Standards 8–14). Within this framework, there are three types of standards of varying stringency: mandates, guidelines, and recommendations as follows:

CLAS mandates are current Federal requirements for all recipients of Federal funds (Standards 4, 5, 6, and 7).

CLAS guidelines are activities recommended by OMH [Office of Minority Health] for adoption as mandates by Federal, State, and national accrediting agencies (Standards 1, 2, 3, 8, 9, 10, 11, 12, and 13).

CLAS recommendations are suggested by OMH for voluntary adoption by healthcare organizations (Standard 14).

Standard 1
Healthcare organizations should ensure that patients/consumers receive from all staff members effective, understandable, and respectful care that is provided in a manner compatible with their cultural health beliefs and practices and preferred language.

Standard 2
Healthcare organizations should implement strategies to recruit, retain, and promote at all levels of the organization a diverse staff and leadership that are representative of the demographic characteristics of the service area.

Standard 3
Healthcare organizations should ensure that staff at all levels and across all disciplines receive ongoing education and training in culturally and linguistically appropriate service delivery.

Continued

Standard 4
Healthcare organizations must offer and provide language assistance services, including bilingual staff and interpreter services, at no cost to each patient/consumer with limited English proficiency at all points of contact, in a timely manner during all hours of operation.

Standard 5
Healthcare organizations must provide to patients/consumers in their preferred language both verbal offers and written notices informing them of their right to receive language assistance services.

Standard 6
Healthcare organizations must assure the competence of language assistance provided to limited English proficient patients/consumers by interpreters and bilingual staff. Family and friends should not be used to provide interpretation services (except on request by the patient/consumer).

Standard 7
Healthcare organizations must make available easily understood patient-related materials and post signage in the languages of the commonly encountered groups and/or groups represented in the service area.

Standard 8
Healthcare organizations should develop, implement, and promote a written strategic plan that outlines clear goals, policies, operational plans, and management accountability/oversight mechanisms to provide culturally and linguistically appropriate services.

Standard 9
Healthcare organizations should conduct initial and ongoing organizational self-assessments of CLAS-related activities and are encouraged to integrate cultural and linguistic competence-related measures into their internal audits, performance improvement programs, patient satisfaction assessments, and outcomes-based evaluations.

Standard 10
Healthcare organizations should ensure that data on the individual patient's/consumer's race, ethnicity, and spoken and written language are collected in health records, integrated into the organization's management information systems, and periodically updated.

Standard 11

Healthcare organizations should maintain a current demographic, cultural, and epidemiological profile of the community as well as a needs assessment to accurately plan for and implement services that respond to the cultural and linguistic characteristics of the service area.

Standard 12

Healthcare organizations should develop participatory, collaborative partnerships with communities and utilize a variety of formal and informal mechanisms to facilitate community and patient/consumer involvement in designing and implementing CLAS-related activities.

Standard 13

Healthcare organizations should ensure that conflict and grievance resolution processes are culturally and linguistically sensitive and capable of identifying, preventing, and resolving cross-cultural conflicts or complaints by patients/consumers.

Standard 14

Healthcare organizations are encouraged to regularly make available to the public information about their progress and successful innovations in implementing the CLAS standards and to provide public notice in their communities about the availability of this information.

Source: U.S. Department of Health and Human Services, the Office of Minority Health.

for all organizations that receive federal funds, such as from Medicaid and Medicare (The Office of Minority Health, 2010). Interpretation services include using certified medical interpreters, healthcare system provided interpreters, or telephone interpretation services. Box 9.3 highlights approaches to interpreter services.

Even with interpreters, it may be difficult for LEP patients to follow instructions when they do not understand the meaning and cultural context of messages. A patient with LEP or poor health literacy may be too embarrassed to admit that she does not understand the APRN's explanation about a medication. Medication labels may be particularly confusing even if they are written in a patient's native language. In addition, some immigrants are not

Box 9.3 Guidelines when using an interpreter

- Use interpreter services or bilingual providers for patients with limited English proficiency.
- Unless thoroughly effective and fluent in the target language, use an interpreter.
- Try to use an interpreter of the same gender as the patient.
- Avoid using family members as interpreters.
  - Children often lack an understanding of health words and issues in either their native language or English.
  - Serving as an interpreter may give children in some cultures more status.
- Learn basic words and sentences in the target language.
- Emphasize important information by repetition.
- Speak slowly and clearly, but not loudly. Do not shout. This does not help the patient or family understand any better.
- Be patient.
- Careful interpretation often requires that long explanatory phrases be used.
- Address the patient directly. Do not direct commentary to the interpreter as if the patient does not exist. Return to an issue if a problem is suspected.
- Be sure the interpreter knows what everyone involved wants.
- Provide instructions in list format and have patients repeat their understanding of medical therapy.
- Use short questions and comments.
- Greet the family with respect; be polite and formal.
- Use simple sentences; keep questions short.
- Use common words in lay terms.
- If it is necessary to use medical jargon, carefully explain it.
- Use 3 × 5-in. language cards with basic phrases spoken by the majority of patients.
- Use picture cards as appropriate.
- Recognize when families may be saying yes, even though they may not understand.
- Avoid technical terminology and professional jargon, like "workup."
- Use language that the interpreter can handle.
- Do not confuse the interpreter by rephasing or hesitating.
- Avoid abstractions, idiomatic expressions, similes, and metaphors.
- Plan what to say ahead of time.

Sources: Lehna, 2005; Muñoz & Luckmann, 2005; Nailon, 2006.

literate in their native language and unable to read any kind of instruction.

Native English language speakers may also need additional support with verbal and written information about medications so the treatment is clearly understood. Patients may have difficulty communicating with their APRN because of low literacy related to learning disorders, poor vision, and lack of education. For example, the directions about daily use of an inhaler for asthma along with an as-needed "rescue" inhaler may be difficult to understand. People who are illiterate often hide their inability to read. This affects their ability to understand written directions for use of medications and can lead to adverse effects or render the medication ineffective. This problem may be identified and addressed if all patients are asked to "read back" the APRN's written instructions.

Both LEP and low literacy may contribute to major health and legal problems. Prescriptions may not be purchased if medication recommendations and their importance are not understood. LEP patients are four times more likely than native English-speaking patients to misunderstand prescriptions when treated by providers who speak a different language from themselves (Wilson, Chen, Grumbach, Wang, & Fernandez, 2005).

Culturally competent communication can promote the right patient using the right prescription in the right way. For some cultural groups, patient education about oral contraceptive pills should clearly specify that the woman, rather than the man, be the one to use the medication. What often seems obvious to APRNs may not be obvious to patients they serve.

It is also important for APRNs to not assume that the patient and family understand the route of administration of a medication. For example, parents may need guidance that an oral antibiotic solution for an ear infection should be taken by mouth rather than being put into the painful ear canal. A poultice or topical gel could mistakenly be eaten rather than applied to the affected skin. A woman may misunderstand the phrase contraceptive gel and assume the provider recommends food-based jelly instead of a contraceptive gel from the pharmacy. One approach to communicate clearly and prevent medication errors is for APRNs to provide a written summary of medication instructions if the patient is literate.

Prescribing for people with disabilities

It is also important to remember that people with disabilities are considered a culture group. It can be challenging to communicate clearly with patients who have visual and hearing impairments. Disabilities may affect access to transportation, financial stability, and social support, and contribute to difficulties in obtaining and using prescriptions. Patients with a speech disability may be unable to communicate their medication history and allergies or to express understanding about the medications prescribed. Strategies to improve communication include: written instructions, pictures and illustrations, hand gestures, and speaking slowly and in a low tone voice. Directly facing the patient, especially in situations where in-room computers are used, allows patients to better hear the APRN and read lips when appropriate.

CULTURE AND THE DYNAMICS OF PRESCRIPTION MEDICATIONS

Many herbs and teas are used as home remedies. For example, boiled peanut root tea, teas containing cedar, cumin, chamomile, spearmint, strawberry, peppermint, cinnamon, and Mormon tea may be used for diarrhea. Boiled chicken fat may be rubbed over the sinuses for an upper respiratory infection. Folk remedies, herbal preparations, and home remedies may interact with prescription medications (National Center for Complementary and Alternative Medicine, 2010). Common examples are listed in Box 9.4.

Prescribing medications in a manner consistent with cultural practices can facilitate their use. In some Asian or Native American cultures, poultices are used more often than oral treatments. A prescription for an ointment, cream, or gel for local analgesia or a skin infection may be better accepted than an oral systemic medication. If, for example, a Chinese American patient uses ginseng tea as a daily treatment, it may be useful to recommend that medication be taken at the same time.

Complementary, alternative, and traditional healthcare treatments

Many cultural groups embrace the use of folk practices, complementary, and alternative therapies, and non-Food and Drug

---

Box 9.4 Herbs and remedies that may interact with medications

1. St. John's wort (*Hypericum perforatum*) for depression
   St. John's wort may cause gastrointestinal disturbances. If taken with nonsteroidal anti-inflammatory drugs (NSAIDs), it can cause gastrointestinal bleeding.
2. Ginkgo biloba taken as an antioxidant
   Ginko biloba has potential interactions with garlic, vitamin E, and medications with antiplatelet or anticoagulant properties.
3. Valerian for sedation in anxiety and restlessness
   Valerian can heighten the effects of anxiolytics, antidepressants, muscle relaxants, and sedatives.

Source: National Center for Complementary and Alternative Medicine, 2010.

Administration-approved medications. Examples of these include acupuncture, Reiki and homeopathic, naturopathic and Chinese herbal medicines. Some Latinos may use botanicals in place of allopathic medicines. Often, a folk healer recommends these treatments. Also, rather than seeking care from an allopathic healer, Latinos may utilize a farmacia or yerberia (e.g., a Mexican-style pharmacy or drugstore) to self-treat or receive advice from an herbalist, pharmacist, or knowledgeable layperson (Spector, 2009) (Fig. 9.1).

The collection of treatments known in the United States as complementary and alternative medicine (CAM) may be viewed as mainstream in many cultures. Allopathic health care may be used by some cultures only when folk practices and CAM fail. Consequently, some patients may be reluctant to seek medications or care from an APRN or to use prescription medications.

In some instances, folk healers may treat as well as refer patients to the APRN for allopathic care. Folk healers may suggest, recommend, or give patients medicines or herbs. APRN collaboration with these healers may promote more effective prescribing. One study about Navajo native healers noted little conflict between

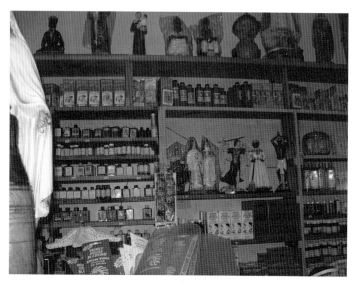

Fig. 9.1 Interior of a Botanica in Boston. Botanicas are Hispanic pharmacies where people are able to purchase traditional herbal remedies, amulets, and statues of saints. They are patronized by people from Mexico, Puerto Rico, and other Hispanic nations. Courtesy of Rachel E. Spector, 2010. Reprinted with permission.

native healers' and allopathic providers' advice (Kim & Kwok, 1998).

Curanderos are highly respected folk healers in Mexican American communities as devout people with extremely religious convictions and acknowledged experts in diagnosing and treating folk illnesses. The *yerbero* is a herbalist who has extensive knowledge about plants and their healing properties; prescribes and prepares herbs, teas, and roots for preventing or curing illnesses; and offers advice on home remedies (Perrone, Stockel, & Krueger, 1989). A *sobador* is similar to a massage therapist or chiropractor and treats illnesses primarily affecting the joints and musculoskeletal system by using massage and manipulation (Perrone et al., 1989). A *parterna* is a lay midwife who treats pregnant women and young children (Perrone et al., 1989).

STRATEGIES FOR PRESCRIBING IN A CULTURALLY COMPETENT MANNER

Prescription medication use and acceptability of a type of medication is influenced by the patient's background and cultural beliefs (Uiters et al., 2006). For example, if prescription and over-the-counter medications are believed to be "too strong," patients may use a lower than prescribed dose. Certain side effects may be particularly troubling such as impotence or diarrhea which may threaten a Latino's sense of manliness (Sobralske, 2006). Some patients believe that drugs should only be administered by injection to be effective. In this situation, the APRN might choose an intramuscular injection of long-acting Bicillin (penicillin) for streptococcal pharyngitis rather than prescribing a 10-day course of oral penicillin.

Since poultices are commonly used in many countries, immigrant parents of a child may mistakenly use an oral suspension antibiotic on an infected wound instead of administering it orally (Galanti, 2008). An immigrant from Asia who typically boils herbs to drink as a single dose will require specific education about the approach of taking medication over a period of time, for example, a 10-day course of oral antibiotics.

APRNs need to build trust with patients so they disclose all their medications, supplements, and treatments. Respect for the patient's choices is important and should be incorporated into prescribing decisions. Simultaneously, the APRN needs to be alert to potential interactions between prescribed medications and CAM therapies.

Another strategy for prescribing in a culturally competent manner is to discuss the patient's explanatory models for a particular condition being treated and understand the cultural meaning of the condition. There may be a word or concept for that condition, such as *malojo* (evil eye) or *susto* (fright sickness), that may not fit into the Westernized concept of illness.

Culturally appropriate education might include additional written instructions about prescribed medications signed by the APRN, to improve understanding in patients from diverse communities. Verification of how the patient will take the medication can be obtained by asking the patient to verbalize understanding of the APRN's instructions.

Box 9.5 Strategies to promote medication use

- Contact social workers or care managers to obtain medications through drug assistance programs and charitable organizations.
- Prescribe less expensive medications if appropriate.
- Select generic medications when available.
- Refer to pharmacies that will mail or deliver medications, if transportation is limited.
- Recommend mail-order pharmacies if they are less expensive than local pharmacies.
- Mail-order pharmacies are an option for people who use long-term medications.
- Recommend pharmacies that have specific low-cost prescription programs.

Source: Compiled from Leonard, 2007.

Sociocultural and economic factors may limit a person's ability to access and use medications. These factors affect vulnerable populations including people who live in poverty or are homeless, as well as people who are underinsured and uninsured. One study found patients from ethnic and racial minority groups spend less money on and use fewer prescription medications than Caucasian patients (Gaskin, Briesacher, Limcangco, & Brigantti, 2006). Many older patients are unable to afford medications despite the Medicare Part D prescription drug program. Box 9.5 includes strategies to promote successful access to and use of medications.

SUMMARY

Quality of patient care can be enhanced by culturally competent prescribing. APRNs have distinguished themselves by using a holistic approach to health care. Consideration of a patient's culture, race, and ethnicity when making prescribing decisions is integral to APRN practice. Cultural competence in advanced nursing practice requires the ability to interact effectively with people of different cultures. Strategies that enhance concordance between the APRN's prescribing approach and the patient's desires and expectations is critical for patient-centered, culturally appropriate care for diverse populations.

REFERENCES

American Anthropological Association. (1997). American anthropological association response to OMB directive 15: Race and ethnic standards for federal statistics and administrative reporting. Retrieved from http://www.aaanet.org/gvt/ombdraft.htm

American Anthropological Association. (2011). About race: A public education project. Retrieved from http://www.aaanet.org/resources/A-Public-Education-Program.cfm

Andrews, M. M. (2007). Cultural diversity and community health nursing. In M. A. Nies, & M. McEwan (Eds.), *Community and public health nursing* (4th ed., pp. 205–235). St. Louis, MO: Elsevier.

Andrews, M. M., & Boyle, J. S. (2008). *Transcultural concepts in nursing care* (5th ed.). Philadelphia: Lippincott, Williams, & Wilkins.

Carey, W. D. (Ed.). (2010). *Cleveland clinic: Current clinical medicine* (2nd ed.). Philadelphia: Saunders Elsevier.

Chaudhry, I. B., Neelam, K., Duddu, V., & Husain, N. (2008). Ethnicity and psychopharmacology. *Journal of Psychopharmacology, 22*(6), 673–680.

Clark, L., & Hofsess, L. (1998). Acculturation. In S. Loue (Ed.), *Handbook of immigrant health* (pp. 37–59). New York: Plenum Press.

Culture Care Connection. (2010). Hmong in Minnesota: Increasing the cultural competence of health care providers serving diverse populations. Retrieved from http://www.culturecareconnection.org/matters/diversity/hmong.html

DeBaun, M. R., & Vichinsky, E. (2007). Hemoglobinopathies. In R. M. Kliegman, R. E. Behrman, H. B. Jenson, & B. F. Stanton (Eds.), *Nelson textbook of pediatrics* (18th ed., pp. 2025–2039). Philadelphia: Saunders Elsevier.

Douglas, J. G., Bakris, G. L., Epstein, M., Ferdinand, K. C., Ferrario, C. Flack, J. M., . . . Vidt, D. G. (2003). Management of high blood pressure in African Americans. Consensus statement of the Hypertension in African Americans Working Group of the International Society of Hypertension in Blacks. *Archives in Internal Medicine, 163*(5), 524–541.

Enattah, N. S., Sahi, T., Savilahti, E., Terwillerger, J. D., Peltonen, L., & Jarvela, I. (2002). Identification of a variant associated with adult-type hypolactasia. *Nature Genetics, 30*(2), 233–237.

Fahrenwald, N. L., Boysen, R., Fischer, C., & Maurer, R. (2001). Developing cultural competence in the baccalaureate nursing student: A population-based project with the Hutterites. *Journal of Transcultural Nursing*, *12*(1), 48–55.

Flack, J. M., Sica, D. A., Bakris, G., Brown, A. L., Ferdinand, K. C., Grimm, R. H. Jr., . . . Jamerson, K. A., on behalf of the International Society on Hypertension in Blacks. (2010). Management of high blood pressure in blacks: An update of the International Society on Hypertension in Blacks consensus statement. *Hypertension*, *56*(5), 780–800.

Franciosa, J. A., Ferdinand, K. C., Yancy, C. W., & Consensus Statement on Heart Failure in African Americans Writing Group. (2010a). Treatment of heart failure in African Americans: A consensus statement. *Congestive Heart Failure*, *16*(1), 27–38.

Franciosa, J. A., Ferdinand, K. C., & Yancy, C. W. (2010b). Treatment of heart failure in African Americans: Executive summary. *Congestive Heart Failure*, *16*(1), 1–2.

Furberg, C. D., Wright, J. T., Davis, B. R., Cutler, J. A., Alderman, M., Black, H., & Pelosi, J. (2002). Major outcomes in high-risk hypertensive patients randomized to angiotensin-converting enzyme inhibitor or calcium channel blocker vs. diuretic: The antihypertensive and lipid-lowering treatment to prevent heart attack trial (ALLHAT). *JAMA*, *288*(23), 2981–2997.

Galanti, G. (2008). *Caring for patients from different cultures* (4th ed.). Philadelphia: University of Pennsylvania Press.

Galanti, G. A. (2004). Basic concepts. In G. A. Galanti (Ed.), *Caring for patients from different cultures* (3rd ed., pp. 1–19). Philadelphia: University of Pennsylvania Press.

Gamble, V. N. (1997). Under the shadow of Tuskegee: African Americans and health care. *American Journal of Public Health*, *87*(11), 1773–1778.

Gaskin, D. J., Briesacher, B. A., Limcangco, R., & Brigantti, B. L. (2006). Exploring racial and ethnic disparities in prescription drug spending and use among Medicare beneficiaries. *American Journal of Geriatric Pharmacotherapeutics*, *4*(2), 93–95.

Giardina, P. J., & Forget, B. G. (2008). Thalassemia syndromes. In R. Hoffman, E. J. Benz, S. J. Shattil, B. Furie, L. E. Silberstein, P. Mc Glave, & H. Helsop (Eds.), *Hematology: Basic principles and practice* (5th ed.). Philadelphia: Elsevier Churchill Livingstone.

Glazer, W. M., (1994). Race and tardive dyskinesia among outpatients at a CMHC. *Hospital Community Psychiatry, 45*(1), 38–42.

Greer, T. M. (2010). Perceived racial discrimination in clinical encounters among African American hypertensive patients. *Journal of Health Care for the Poor and Underserved, 21*(1), 251–263.

Gupta, A. K., Poulter, N. R., Dobson, J., Eldridge, S., Cappuccio, F. P., Caufield, M., . . . Feder, G. (2010). Ethnic differences in blood pressure responses to first and second-line antihypertensive therapies in patients randomized in the ASCOT Trial. *American Journal of Hypertension, 23*(9), 1023–1030.

Hamilton, J. A. (2008). Revitalizing difference in the HapMap: Race and contemporary human genetic variation research. *Journal of Law and Medical Ethics, 36*(3), 471–477.

Harmon, A. (2010, April 21). Indian tribe wins fight to limit research of its DNA. *The New York Times*, p. A1.

Johnson, J. A. (2008). Ethnic differences in cardiovascular drug response: Potential contribution of pharmacogenetics. *Circulation, 118*(13), 1383–1393.

Kataoka-Yahiro, M., Ceria, C., & Caulfield, R. (2004). Grandparents' caregiving role in ethnically diverse families. *Journal of Pediatric Nursing, 19*(5), 315–328.

Kim, C., & Kwok, Y. S. (1998). Navajo use of native healers. *Archive of Internal Medicine, 158*(20), 2245–2249.

Kleinman, A. (1980). *Patients and healers in the context of culture.* Berkeley, CA: University of California Press.

Lehna, C. (2005). Interpreter services in pediatric nursing. *Pediatric Nursing, 31*(4), 292–296.

Leininger, M. M., & McFarland, M. (2006). *Culture care diversity and universality: A worldwide nursing theory* (2nd ed.). Sudbury, MA: Jones & Bartlett.

Leonard, K. (2007). Cultural competency: An outside the box perspective. The Lancet Student. Retrieved from http://www.thelancetstudent.com/2007/10/03/cultural-competency-an-outside-the-box-perspective/

Mangravite, L. M., Wilke, R. A., Zhang, J., & Krauss, R. M. (2008). Pharmacogenomics of statin response. *Current Opinion in Molecular Therapeutics, 10*(6), 555–561.

Meyer, J. M., Rosenblatt, L., Kim, E., Baker, R. A., & Whitehead, R. (2009). The moderating impact of ethnicity on metabolic outcomes with olanzapine and aripiprazole in patients with schizophrenia. *Journal of Clinical Psychiatry*, *70*(3), 318–325.

Muñoz, C. C., & Hilgenberg, C. (2005). Ethnopharmacology. *American Journal of Nursing*, *105*(8), 40–48.

Muñoz, C. C., & Luckmann, J. (2005). *Transcultural communication in nursing* (2nd ed.). Clifton Park, NY: Thomson/Delmar Learning.

Nailon, R. E. (2006). Nurses' concerns and practices with using interpreters in the care of Latino patients in the emergency department. *Journal of Transcultural Nursing*, *17*(2), 119–128.

National Center for Complementary and Alternative Medicine. (2010). Herbs at a glance. Retrieved from http://nccam.nih.gov/health/valerian

Neff, N. (1999). Module VII: Folk medicine in Hispanics in the Southwestern United States. Retrieved from http://www.rice.edu/projects/HispanicHealth/Courses/mod7/mod7.html

Norris, K. C., Tareen, N., Martins, D., & Vaziri, N. D. (2008). Implications of ethnicity for the treatment of hypertensive kidney disease, with an emphasis on African Americans. *Nature Reviews Nephrology*, *4*(10), 538–549.

Ogedegbe, G., Mancuso, C. A., & Allegrante, J. P. (2004). Expectations of blood pressure management in hypertensive African-American patients: A qualitative study. *Journal of the National Medical Association.*, *96*, 442–449.

Olfsun, M., & Marcus, S. C. (2009). National patterns in antidepressant medication treatment. *Archives of General Psychiatry*, *66*(8), 848–856.

O'Loughlin, J., Dugas, E., Maximova, K., & Kishchuk, N. (2006). Reporting of ethnicity in research on chronic disease: Update. *Postgraduate Medical Journal*, *82*(973), 737–742.

Ortiz, B. I., Shields, K. M., Clauson, K. A., & Clay, P. G. (2007). Complementary and alternative medicine use among Hispanics in the United States. *Annals of Pharmacotherapy*, *41*(6), 994–1004.

Perrone, B., Stockel, H. H., & Krueger, V. (1989). *Medicine women, curanderas, and women doctors*. Norman, OK: University of Oklahoma Press.

Roger, V. L., Go, A. S., Lloyd-Jones, D. M., Adams, R. J., Berry, J. D., Brown, T. M., . . . Wylie-Rosett, J. (2011). Heart disease and stroke statistics 2011 update: A report from the American Heart Association. Retrieved from http://circ.ahajournals.org/cgi/content/full/123/4/e18?maxtoshow=&hits=10&RESULTFORMAT=&fulltext=heaRT+DISEASE+ANDSTROKE+STATISTICS+2011&searchid=1&FIRSTINDEX=0&resourcetype=HWCIT

Sobralske, M. C. (2006). Health care seeking among Mexican American men. *Journal of Transcultural Nursing, 17*(2), 129–138.

Spector, R. E. (2009). *Cultural diversity in health and illness* (7th ed.). Upper Saddle River, NJ: Pearson, Prentice Hall.

Teal, C. R., & Street, R. L. (2009). Critical elements of culturally competent communication in the medical encounter: A review and model. *Social Sciences & Medicine, 68*(3), 533–543.

The Office of Minority Health, United States. (2010). National standards on culturally and linguistically appropriate services. Department of Health and Human Services. Retrieved from http://minorityhealth.hhs.gov/templates/browse.aspx?lvl=2&lvlID=15

Turner, B. J., Hollenbeak, C., Weiner, M. G., Ten Have, T., & Roberts, C. (2009). Barriers to adherence and hypertension control in a racially diverse representative sample of elderly primary care patients. *Pharmacoepidemiology and Drug Safety, 18*(8), 672–681.

Uiters, E., van Dijk, L., Deville, W., Foets, M., Spreeuwenberg, P., & Groenewegen, P. P. (2006). Ethnic minorities and prescription medications: Concordance between self-reports and medical records. *BMC Health Services Research, 6*(115), 1–7.

Wilson, E., Chen A., H., Grumbach, K., Wang, F., & Fernandez, A. (2005). Effects of limited English proficiency and physician language on health care comprehension. *Journal of General Internal Medicine, 20*(9), 800–806.

Links to web-based resources

The Center for Cross-Cultural Health, http://www.caringcommunity.org/node/view/361

The Cross Cultural Health Care Program, www.xculture.org

Cultural Competence website, http://cecp.air.org/cultural/

Cultural Competency Standards http://www.omhrc.gov/clas/indexfinal.htm

Diversity Rx, www.diversityrx.org

EthnoMED, http://ethnomed.org/

Health Resources and Services Administration. Cultural Competence Resources for Health Care Providers, http://www.hrsa.gov/culturalcompetence/

National Center for Cultural Competence, http://www11.georgetown.edu/research/gucchd/nccc/

The Office of Minority Health, http://minorityhealth.hhs.gov/

The Process of Cultural Competence in the Delivery of Health care Services, http://www.transculturalcare.net/Cultural_Competence_Model.htm

Transcultural C.A.R.E Associates, www.transculturalcare.net

Transcultural Nursing Society, www.tcns.org

Index

Page numbers in *italics* refer to figures; those in **boldface**, tables.

The Advanced Practice Registered Nurse as a Prescriber, First Edition. Marie Annette
Brown, Louise Kaplan.
© 2012 John Wiley & Sons, Ltd. Published 2012 by John Wiley & Sons, Ltd.